The Jossey-Bass/AHA Press Series translates the latest ideas on health care management into practical and actionable terms. Together, Jossey-Bass and the American Hospital Association offer these essential resources for the health care leaders of today and tomorrow.

Changing Patient Behavior

Richard Patterson, Editor

. . . .

Changing Patient Behavior

. . . .

Improving Outcomes in Health and Disease Management

WITHDRAWN

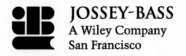

JOSSEY-BASS
A Wiley Company
San Francisco

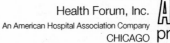

Health Forum, Inc.
An American Hospital Association Company
CHICAGO press

Jossey-Bass books and products are available through most bookstores. To contact Jossey-Bass directly, call (888) 378-2537, fax to (800) 605-2665, or visit our website at www.josseybass.com.

Substantial discounts on bulk quantities of Jossey-Bass books are available to corporations, professional associations, and other organizations. For details and discount information, contact the special sales department at Jossey-Bass.

Library of Congress Cataloging-in-Publication Data

Changing patient behavior : improving outcomes in health and disease management / Richard Patterson, editor.
     p. cm. —(The Jossey-Bass/AHA Press series)
Includes bibliographical references and index.
    ISBN 0-7879-5279-6 (alk. paper)
  1. Disease management. 2. Behavior therapy. 3. Outcome assessment (Medical care) I. Patterson, Richard, 1957– II. Series.
    RA394 .C46 2001
    615.5'071—dc21   00-010153

Contents

· ·

List of Exhibits, Figures, and Tables

. . . .

Tables

About the Authors

. . . .

L. Kay Bartholomew, Ed.D., M.P.H., is associate director of the Center for Health Promotion and Prevention Research at the University of Texas Health Science Center in Houston. She serves as associate professor of behavioral sciences in the School of Public Health. She has worked in the field of health education and health promotion since her graduation from Austin College more than twenty-five years ago, first at a city-county health department and later at Texas Children's Hospital. Currently, in her research center and faculty roles she teaches courses in health promotion intervention development and conducts research in chronic disease self-management. Dr. Bartholomew received her M.P.H. from the University of Texas–Houston School of Public Health and her Ed.D. from the University of Houston College of Education. She has won the Society for Public Health Education Program Excellence Award for the Cystic Fibrosis Family Education Program as well as numerous other professional association and media awards.

Joseph E. Biskupiak, Ph.D., M.B.A., is therapeutics strategist for EMA Strategic Consulting, Somerville, New Jersey, a subsidiary of Skila Inc., Mahwah, New Jersey. He is a strategic consultant to the pharmaceutical and medical device industries. Prior to joining Skila, he was vice president of health services research at Hastings Healthcare Group in Pennington, New Jersey. In addition, he was a research assistant professor in the Office of Health Policy and Clinical Outcomes at Thomas Jefferson University Hospital in Philadelphia. He was also a research scientist and research assistant professor in the Department of Radiology at the University of Washington School of Medicine in Seattle and a research investigator at E. R. Squibb and Sons. Dr. Biskupiak has published widely, particularly in the basic and applied sciences and health services research field. He contributed the chapters "Disease Management Programs" in the textbook *The Role of Pharmacoeconomics in Outcomes Management* and "Managed Care Models of Disease Management" in *Disease Management: A Systems Approach to Improving Patient Outcomes*, both 1996 publications of AHA Press. He earned a Ph.D. in medicinal chemistry from the University of Utah, an M.B.A. from Seattle University, and a B.S. in chemistry from the University of Connecticut.

Celeste Cafiero, M.A., C.H.E.S., is vice president of consumer content for HealthAnswers.com in Pennington, New Jersey. She is responsible for development of consumer education and disease management features on the web site. Previously, she was vice president of outcomes management for Hastings Healthcare Group and created programs to enhance compliance with medical and lifestyle treatment plans. Prior to that, she was editor-in-chief, consumer health, for Mosby-Wolfe Medical Communications, overseeing product development of all disease management and patient support programs for Mosby's pharmaceutical accounts worldwide. Before joining Mosby, she was vice president of product development for Great Performance, Inc., a health care communications company. Ms. Cafiero's program management experience is drawn from having directed nationwide health promotion activities for clients of The Prudential Group Department and having designed, managed, and evaluated Metropolitan Life Insurance Company's original employee worksite risk reduction program. She has been involved in the areas of health education and communications for the past twenty years.

Fern Carness, M.P.H., R.N., C.C.R.N., is principal of Carness Health Management, LLC, a health management consulting firm located in Portland, Oregon. She is a well-respected, highly acclaimed health professional with twenty-five years' experience in health care delivery, health education, behavior change, worksite health promotion, interactive program design, and population health management. Ms. Carness is a nationally known speaker, trainer, and author. Publications include the highly effective *Ready Set STOP!*, *How to Quit Quitting,* and *Wise Woman's Approach to Healing and Cancer.* She has created strategies to support NCQA/HEDIS compliance and directed the development of disease-state management programs in a pharmaceutical benefits management environment. Programming she has developed, directed, and coordinated includes telephony triage, medical self-care, clinical evaluations, disease management, medical and behavioral interventions, case management, patient education, demand management, health risk and other assessments, and member awareness programs.

Karen Glanz, Ph.D., M.P.H., is a professor in the Prevention and Control Program at the Cancer Research Center of Hawaii, University of Hawaii at Manoa, in Honolulu. She previously was a professor in the Department of Health Education at Temple University in Philadelphia, an adjunct professor in the Temple University School of Medicine, and an adjunct member at Fox Chase Cancer Center. Her research interests have been the determinants of health-related behavior, patient education, nutrition behavior and education, and cancer prevention and control. She was lead editor of the book *Health Behavior and Health Education: Theory, Research, and Practice* (Jossey-Bass, 1990 and 1997) and was co-recipient (with Frances Lewis and Barbara Rimer) of the Mayhew

Derryberry Award for outstanding contributions to theory and research in health education from the Public Health Education and Health Promotion Section of the American Public Health Association.

Nell H. Gottlieb, Ph.D., is professor and coordinator of health education programs in the Department of Kinesiology and Health Education at the University of Texas at Austin and professor of behavioral science at the University of Texas–Houston School of Public Health. She received her Ph.D. in sociology from Boston University. She is author of numerous articles and two textbooks. Her interests are in multilevel health promotion intervention development and evaluation, particularly in the area of tobacco prevention and control. Dr. Gottlieb has served as chair of the Health Education and Promotion Section of the American Public Health Association and as the president of the Society for Public Health Education.

Gerjo Kok, Ph.D., is dean of the School of Psychology at Maastricht University in the Netherlands and is professor of applied psychology. From 1984 to 1998 he was professor of health education and chair of the Department of Health Education at Maastricht University. He holds the endowed chair for AIDS Prevention and Health Promotion of the Dutch AIDS Fund. Dr. Kok received his Ph.D. in social psychology at Groningen University. He has extensive publications in the areas of social psychology and health.

Terry Mason, M.P.H., develops and evaluates health and disease management programs. She has developed programs for managed care organizations, industry, and the Internet and has consulted for companies worldwide. She was director of development for American Corporate Health Programs, Inc., and Johnson & Johnson Advanced Behavioral Technologies. She develops high-risk and disease management programs that use the Internet, telephone, mail, and interactive voice response systems. Ms. Mason is the author of many articles and has spoken nationally and internationally on reaching dispersed and targeted populations with health programming.

Daniel L. Newton, Ph.D., M.S., is president of The NewSof Group, Inc., a Seattle-based consulting company focused on the application of technology for health-related strategies and program development. He was a team leader within Monsanto responsible for the initial concept development of Lexant prior to becoming a vice president and corporate officer for Lexant, a technology-centered population health services company that delivers behaviorally based disease and lifestyle management interventions. Before joining Lexant, he was a senior consultant with The Benfield Group, a national health care consulting firm specializing in the strategic analysis, development, and evaluation of health and wellness business opportunities. He has over fifteen years' experience in the various areas of health risk management ranging from cost-benefit research to building entrepreneurial ventures in health management–related businesses. He has directed extensive research on the economic impact of worksite health promotion while at The American University's National Center for Health/Fitness, spoken at national and international forums, and has been active in developing integrated approaches for assessing, monitoring, and measuring population health risks. As COO for an international joint-venture company focused on diversified human resource services, he designed and developed comprehensive health and worklife programs for large health care, corporate, and government institutions. He also developed information and software systems to support outcomes measurement and developed specific health risk intervention programs for commercial and corporate distribution. Dr. Newton has been recognized and commended by the U.S.

Army Materiel Command, the National Center for Health/Fitness, and The American University for his contributions relating to health promotion. He has a Ph.D. in educational administration and an M.S. in health/fitness management from The American University.

Brian Oldenburg, Ph.D., M.Psychol., is professor and head of school at the School for Public Health at the Queensland University of Technology in Queensland, Australia. From 1994 to 1998 he was also the director for the Centre for Public Health Research. He is the regional editor of the international journal *Psychology and Health* and the president-elect of the International Society for Behavioral Medicine. He is a past president of the Division of Health Psychology, International Association of Applied Psychology. He is a clinical health psychologist who has been researching public health issues for more than twenty years, with particular interest in developing, implementing, and evaluating public health interventions in a range of settings, including primary health care, the workplace, and schools. His particular areas of interest include cardiovascular risk reduction and sociobehavioral epidemiology.

Guy S. Parcel, Ph.D., John P. McGovern professor of health promotion, is director of the Center for Health Promotion and Prevention Research at the University of Texas Health Science Center in Houston. He serves as professor of behavioral sciences and associate dean for research in the School of Public Health. He has directed research projects to develop and evaluate programs to address sexual risk behavior for adolescents, diet and physical activity in children, self-management of childhood chronic diseases, smoking prevention, sun protection for preschool children, and the diffusion of health promotion programs. Dr. Parcel received his B.S. and M.S. degrees in health education at Indiana University and his Ph.D. at Penn State University with a major in health education and a minor in child development and family relations. He has authored or coauthored more than 180 scientific papers and received the American School Health Association 1990 William A. Howe Award for outstanding contributions and distinguished service in school health.

Richard Patterson, M.S., is executive vice president, director of development for HealthAnswers.com, a consumer health information and health management web site. Prior to its acquisition by HealthAnswers, Inc., Mr. Patterson was the founder and managing director of Hastings Outcomes Management, a health management company located in Pennington, New Jersey. Mr. Patterson was an innovator in the commercial application of health-related behavior change principles and message tailoring to the management of people with chronic illnesses. Hastings' programs for people with Parkinson's disease, depression, and arthritis were demonstrated to improve clinical, cost of care, health-related quality of life, and patient satisfaction outcomes through outcomes research studies. Since 1986, Mr. Patterson has led the development of health management interventions in more than a dozen clinical conditions. Mr. Patterson earned M.S. degrees in biological chemistry and human genetics from the University of Michigan at Ann Arbor and a B.S. degree in biochemistry from the State University of New York at Stony Brook. He has been a frequent speaker and author on the subjects of disease management and the applications of health behavior change interventions.

Laura T. Pizzi, Pharm.D., is currently manager of outcomes research at HealthAnswers, Inc., Pennington, New Jersey. She is actively involved in developing and implementing disease management content for the company's consumer web site, HealthAnswers.com. Dr. Pizzi holds a bachelor's degree and a doctorate of pharmacy from Rutgers University College of Pharmacy and is currently pursuing a master's degree in public health at the New Jersey School of Public Health in Piscataway, New Jersey.

Neal S. Sofian, M.S.P.H., is the CEO of The NewSof Group, Inc.,
a Seattle-based consulting company focused on the application of
technology for health-related strategies and program development.
He was the original vice president of Lexant within Monsanto,
responsible for its start-up. Lexant is a technology-centered population health services company that delivers behaviorally based disease and lifestyle management interventions. Prior to starting
Lexant, he was the general manager of Health At Work managing
worksite and community health promotion programs and served as
a manager for innovation for over fourteen years for Group Health
Cooperative of Puget Sound. He directed the development, implementation, and marketing of all health promotion, preventive care,
and disease management services, serving employers, insurers, and
health care organizations throughout the United States and
Canada. He was also responsible for the commercialization of Free
& Clear, the nation's first telephonically based tobacco cessation
program, since used as a model for many other telephonic health
risk and disease management programs. Mr. Sofian is a nationally
known speaker and author on topics ranging from integrating
communication technologies into behavioral interventions, to
population-based tobacco cessation strategies, to the role of humor
as an organizational development tool. Earlier he was assistant
director of the Bureau of Community Health Education in the
Missouri State Division of Health and a clinical instructor in the
Department of Family and Community Medicine, University of
Missouri School of Medicine. He holds a master's degree in public
health from the University of Missouri.

Michael R. Toscani, Pharm.D., is adjunct clinical professor at the
Rutgers University School of Pharmacy and senior vice president–
technology assessment at HealthAnswers, Inc., in Pennington, New
Jersey. His comprehensive work in systems design and implementation of disease management initiatives includes modifying provider
behavior (treatment and diagnostic guidelines and education), value

assessments (claims analysis and pharmacoeconomic modeling), and outcome studies (research design and analysis). He applies strong scientific training in directing and managing a variety of pharmacological research projects on approved and investigational drugs. While in the clinical research and development department of Miles Pharmaceuticals (now Bayer), he participated in the prelaunch and postmarketing phases in the development of anti-infective and cardiovascular products. Dr. Toscani received a doctorate and a bachelor of science in pharmacy from St. John's University College of Pharmacy. He completed a postdoctoral research and teaching fellowship in infectious disease at Hartford Hospital. A frequent national speaker and author in both scientific and health care management circles, he serves on the editorial board of the *Journal of Clinical Outcomes Management*. Formerly he served on the editorial boards of the *Journal of Osteopathic Medicine* and the *Journal of Clinical Research and Pharmacoepidemiology*.

*I would like to dedicate this book to my wife Barbara
and my children Alexa and Ryan,
and thank them for their love and support
and for giving purpose to my life.*

*They provide, after all, the most important
and significant influence on my behavior.*

Foreword

Disease management represents a major transformation of modern medicine. Changes are occurring in almost every aspect of health care: from an emphasis on acute illness to a focus on chronic disease; from acute care to a continuum of care; from the treatment of illness exclusively to a balanced maintenance of wellness; and from a reliance on biology alone to a balanced effort to prevent disease and manage it when it occurs. The search for a multitude of germs and genes that contribute to disease is balanced by a concern about a small range of behavior that is essential to life and health.

Breathing, drinking, eating, and moving are simple processes that sustain our bodies. But when they include cigarettes, alcohol abuse, high-fat diets, or a sedentary lifestyle, they can endanger our well-being. A small number of unhealthy habits account for a high percentage of chronic diseases and health care costs, and changing them can become the behavioral equivalent of life-saving surgery. People are often not prepared to take immediate action to prevent disease. We need especially to learn to reach out to people with high-risk conditions because they typically do not reach out to us for help with these silent killers. Passive-reactive practices can work with acute conditions; patients who are in pain, sick, or in distress come to professionals for help. But to combat the chronic diseases of our time professional practice needs to include proactive approaches in which we reach out to help people at high risk before they become sick and in pain.

The transformation in medicine includes a shift from assuming that health care takes place primarily in hospitals and outpatient practices to an acceptance that much of health care takes place in homes. And the patient is becoming the primary care provider, with health care specialists serving as important members of the patient's team. Just as pharmaceuticals can be prescribed in the office and taken at home, so too can disease management begin in the office or hospital and continue at home. What will be modern behavior medicine's equivalent to pharmaceuticals? One projection is that interactive information technologies will be a cost-effective method for delivering the optimal amount of science to bear on key behavior problems in entire populations in a user friendly manner and with no known side effects.

These are exciting times. These are stressful times. These are times when patients and professionals need to progress through the painful process of changing health-related behavior that has been established over a personal or professional lifetime. Only through such a transformation can health care services catch up to the chronic conditions that have been the primary causes of premature death since early in the twentieth century. Early in the twenty-first century, patients and professionals in partnership must learn to better manage wellness and illness. This book can help lead the way.

James O. Prochaska, Ph.D.   September 2000
Director and Professor
Cancer Prevention Research Center
University of Rhode Island

Changing Patient Behavior

. . . .

The New Focus

Integrating Behavioral Science into Disease Management

Richard Patterson

The concept of disease management (also referred to as *population-based health management*) is receiving a great deal of attention and interest from many sectors of the health care system—managed care, health care providers, product manufacturers, and marketers. But what exactly is disease management? Although consensus is building, there does not appear to be a clear definition to which all parties agree. There are, however, a number of elements that are consistent across most definitions of the term.

Definitions of Disease Management

Nearly all definitions of disease management include the following factors:

- A concern with chronic, as opposed to acute, conditions

- A shift in the treatment of chronic disease from discrete episodes of care to care across the continuum of the condition

- A coordinated effort through an integrated system for delivery of health care services

Following are definitions from several sources. Disease management is

- "An approach to patient care that coordinates medical resources for patients across the entire health care delivery system" (Boston Consulting Group, 1995)

- "An approach to patient care that emphasizes coordinated, comprehensive care along the continuum of disease and across health care delivery systems" (Ellrodt and others, 1997, p. 1687)

- "Information-based processes involving improvement of value in all aspects of care throughout the entire spectrum of health care delivery that attempt to produce the best clinical outcomes in the most cost-effective manner" (Peterson, 1995, p. 39)

- "A systematic post-disease attempt to prevent consequences of that disease with long-term management" (Musich, Burton, and Edington, 1999)

Although there are common elements in these definitions, there is no universally accepted goal of disease management. In fact, disease management goals and definitions are often rooted in the point of view of the observer, which is significantly influenced by environment and enlightened self-interest.

Recently the terms *health management* and *population-based health management* have been favored over *disease management* to widen the focus of the approach from chronic illness management to include certain concepts from demand management, in which preventive measures are used to reduce high-risk individuals' chances of contracting the chronic diseases and conditions in the first place.

The Health Plan's Point of View

For most health plans, interest in disease management stems from three relevant areas:

- The need to contain the rate of cost increase for providing health care services

- The demand by customers to improve both the quality of care and level of service

- The need for accreditation from organizations such as the National Committee for Quality Assurance and the Joint Commission on Accreditation of Healthcare Organizations

Analyses of medical claims and other administrative databases have shown that most health care costs in a population with a chronic illness are incurred by a relatively small percentage of the population. Thus, if patients at high risk of incurring significant cost can be prospectively identified and managed, significant reductions in resource utilization can be effected.

Another important factor in managing chronic diseases is the variability in clinical management. Analysis of two years of claims data on approximately two million lives showed that the majority of patients treated for asthma, diabetes, and congestive heart failure does not receive care recommended in expert guidelines (Medstat Group, 1999). Reducing unexplained variability in clinical practice is a second area of focus for managed care plans.

As a result of these influences, two of the most common disease management tactics employed by health plans are analysis of administrative data to identify high-cost patients and application of clinical guidelines ("Disease Management Strategic Research Study and Resource Guide," 1988).

The Health Care Provider's Point of View

For physicians and other health care providers, disease management is often something that is done *to* them rather than *with* them. Most physicians have learned to rely on their training and direct experience to guide them in managing their patients, and so disease management programs—often accompanied by practice management guidelines, new performance measurements, and education—may be seen as incursions on their territory.

In addition, disease management programs frequently ask health care providers to delve into an area of care in which they are uncomfortable—helping patients change their lifestyles or other behavior. For example, the World Health Organization lists twenty-five diseases associated with smoking, yet fewer than half of smokers report being urged to quit by their physician (Department of Health and Human Services, 1996, p. 3). In an independent study of attitudes of primary care physicians, internists, and cardiologists toward lifestyle change in hypertension patients, approximately 40 percent of respondents (primarily the cardiologists, who tended to treat patients with serious illness) viewed themselves as active managers of the patient's efforts to change lifestyle. Another 45 percent of the respondents felt that it was their role to encourage change, but that the responsibility for change lies with the patient. Important factors cited were lack of time, training, and resources. Finally, approximately 15 percent of the participants expressed the point of view that patients are already aware of the impact of lifestyle on heart disease and the physician is unlikely to have any further influence (Vanderveer Group, 1991).

The Patient's Point of View

Patients who enroll in disease management programs are often asked to make a litany of changes—to give up pleasures like favorite foods, smoking, and alcohol. They are then asked to add inconvenient or unpleasant tasks like taking medications with attendant side effects, undergoing regular monitoring, and starting an exercise program. From the patient's viewpoint, the care received doesn't change much—before the program they saw the doctor every few weeks or months or when they became acutely ill, and they continue to see them on the same schedule. Perhaps they now have access to more information or education or even a case manager if acutely ill. However, the responsibility for care remains with the health care providers, while the burden of executing the care plan to manage the illness remains with the patient.

Shifting the Paradigm: Disease-Centered Versus Patient-Centered Approaches

We all know intuitively and from direct personal experience that we are more likely to follow a path we choose than one imposed on us. However, the current approach to disease management is essentially one where a process is dictated by an organization (health plans) and imposed on the members of the organization (health care providers and patients). In addition, the processes of disease management remain focused on the disease, not the patient with the disease. These are fundamental properties of the disease management paradigm that have a significant impact on the success (or lack thereof) of the process. In a nutshell, the best designed process will fail if nobody follows it.

For health and disease management programs to succeed, the paradigm must shift to make behavior change in both health care provider and patient an integral part of the process.

The Role of Behavior in Preventing and Managing Disease

As we have stated earlier, a fundamental property of health and disease management processes is that they are focused on chronic (as opposed to acute) health issues. For the purposes of health management, the definition of *chronic* needs to include not only lifelong conditions, but also conditions that may be resolved within a fixed but relatively prolonged period. For example, management of women with high-risk pregnancies is often a focus of health management processes, yet pregnancy is clearly not a lifelong condition. Other conditions amenable to disease management that are not necessarily lifelong include allergic rhinitis and depression. Because these processes occur over a relatively prolonged period of time, patient adherence (or compliance) to a management process becomes a significant issue.

A second fundamental property of health and disease management processes is that these processes are designed to manage populations across the continuum of health status, from people without current illness but with significant risk factors through those who have significant disease requiring active and intensive clinical intervention. Preventive and risk-reduction behavior is a key component of managing at-risk populations.

Finally, lifestyle behavior has been shown to be a significant contributor and a primary risk factor for numerous chronic diseases (Prochaska, Redding, and Evers, 1997).

Adherence Behavior

Adherence (often called *compliance* in the past) is actually a complex spectrum of behavior that is in part dependent on the regimen to which the patient is asked to adhere. Although most people think of medication compliance, the term *adherence* is applicable to any behavior in which the outcome is dependent on that behavior occurring on a regular and specific schedule.

Regular or periodic monitoring is a crucial activity for many people with chronic conditions such as diabetes, congestive heart failure, and asthma. For example, daily monitoring of body weight on awakening is an important means of detecting fluid retention in patients with congestive heart failure. Patients who weigh themselves only three days a week as well as those who monitor at different times each day would be considered nonadherent. Each of these patients could miss a potentially deadly fluid buildup.

Another type of adherence behavior is restrictive behavior. For example, patients with congestive heart failure are generally put on a sodium-restricted diet that requires them to adopt a number of new habits, including giving up added table salt and salty snack foods as well as learning to read prepared and packaged food product labels for sodium levels.

The terms *compliance* and *adherence* are most commonly applied to medication-taking behavior. There are several types of nonadherence:

- *Refusal of the patient to comply with a prescribed medication regimen*. This can be expressed as *direct refusal* when the patient tells the physician that he or she does not intend to take the medication. More common is *indirect refusal*—the patient accepts a prescription from the physician but does not get it filled or delivers the prescription to the pharmacy but refuses to pick it up. Several models of health behavior described in this book can be applied to explain and successfully intervene in this type of nonadherence behavior.

- *Partial adherence*, in which patients take some, but not all, of the prescribed doses of medication. This behavior includes patients

  Having difficulty establishing the habit of taking medications at the appropriate frequency or timing

  Choosing to take "medication holidays" on weekends and vacations

  Avoiding taking medications for fear of embarrassment or stigma

  Taking a lower dose of medication to save money or avoid side effects

  Taking medications at higher doses or frequency than prescribed because they believe that if some medication is helpful, more medication is more helpful

• *Premature discontinuation*, in which patients stop taking chronic medications without the knowledge or advice of their physicians. This behavior includes patients

Forgetting to refill a medication and in the absence of direct consequences (symptoms) choosing not to continue treatment

Experiencing uncomfortable side effects and finding it too difficult to continue tolerating treatment

Remaining uncertain or unconvinced of the benefits of treatment and then allowing any inconvenience or barrier to persuade them to discontinue treatment

Preventive Behavior

Preventive behavior reduces the risk of developing or exacerbating a condition and is often the focus of public health initiatives. Examples of preventive behavior are use of safe sex practices to prevent transmission of HIV, frequent hand washing to prevent communication of influenza virus or rhinovirus, and use of seat belts to reduce fatalities in automobile accidents.

Lifestyle Behavior

Lifestyle factors like tobacco use, unhealthy diets, alcohol abuse, sedentary lifestyles, stress, obesity, and chronic hostility contribute to the progression of many chronic illnesses, exacerbate others, and in some cases are considered to be causal factors of disease. Table 1.1 shows lifestyle behavior that significantly contributes to some common diseases.

Behavioral Science—An Attempt to Understand Human Behavior

Jim is fifty-three years old and has had adult onset diabetes for nearly ten years. He has read all of the diabetes booklets and other materials his doctors have given him over the years. He is well aware that

Table 1.1.   Common Diseases with Significant Lifestyle Contributors.

Disease	Tobacco Smoking	Unhealthy Diet	Sedentary Lifestyle	Stress	Obesity
Asthma	√			√	
Anxiety disorder			√	√	
Atopic dermatitis (eczema)				√	
Cancer	√	√	√	√	
Depression			√	√	
Diabetes (Type II)	√	√	√		√
Gastroesophageal reflux disease (GERD)	√	√	√	√	√
Headache			√	√	
Hypertension	√		√	√	√
Irritable bowel syndrome				√	
Psoriasis				√	

the cornerstones of managing his diabetes are taking his medicine every day, quitting smoking, watching what he eats, keeping his weight down, and staying physically active. He also knows that, to keep his blood sugar in control, he needs to regularly monitor his blood glucose. And he understands what the consequences may be if he doesn't take care of himself—loss of vision, limbs, or even his life. Yet with all that knowledge, Jim still smokes a pack of cigarettes a day, is twenty-five pounds overweight, rarely exercises, and doesn't monitor his blood glucose nearly as often as his doctor recommends. Jim feels guilty that he can't seem to stick to his diet as well as he knows he should, and exercise seems to be the first thing eliminated from his schedule whenever he gets busy at work.

Patients like Jim are endlessly frustrating to physicians. Jim understands his condition and the requirements of treatment and knows what could happen if he doesn't follow the doctor's orders. Yet he seems incapable of following his diabetes management plan.

Jim is frustrated as well. When he thinks about his diabetes management, he feels like he has lost control over himself. It makes him feel weak and guilty, rather than the intelligent, strong, capable person he believes himself to be in other areas of his life. So why does Jim find it so hard to do what he knows is in his own best interest?

The contributors to this book have provided the specifics of models of health behavior that can be applied to Jim's situation. Let us use Jim's example to walk through some of the concepts applied in these models.

To begin, managing diabetes is not a single behavior, but a complex set of interrelated types of behavior. As a general rule, the more kinds of behavior you expect someone to change simultaneously, the lower the probability that the person will be able to successfully change or maintain a change to *any* behavior. In Jim's case, he was told he needed to make the following changes simultaneously: quit smoking, eliminate interesting foods from his diet, start a program of regular exercise, begin a regimen of medications with sometimes unpleasant side effects, and monitor his blood glucose by creating a small puncture wound in his finger.

One of the cornerstones of health behavior change is, of course, knowledge. A complementary and often necessary adjunct to knowledge is skill. An important part of Jim's diabetes management routine is monitoring serum glucose. To do this, Jim not only learned how to use the lancet and glucose monitor, but also how to read and interpret the results. In addition, Jim learned how to use the lancet with a minimum of discomfort and without substantial risk of infection. He also had to learn what to do if his glucose was outside the normal range. The cognitive knowledge he gained about the role of serum glucose and devices to measure it would not have had much value without the skills he developed in using the devices, interpreting the results, and applying them to keep his serum glucose within the normal range.

Another factor in behavior change is motivation. How motivated is Jim to make the changes he knows he should? First, let's look at how he deals with his dietary changes. Jim knows that in the future, his diabetes could have some serious consequences. However, he generally feels good—he can do pretty much everything he likes to do without much interference from his health. And for the most part his medicine seems to be doing a good job of keeping his blood glucose levels in the right range (when he takes it as prescribed, which he always does regularly before he has appointments with his doctor). So at home, with his wife's help, Jim is able to manage his diet quite well. At work it's another story. When Jim is busy (which is most of the time), he has to grab a quick bite. The only thing close by is a string of fast food chains—and he really loves french fries. So even though Jim has the motivation to stick to his diet at home, a different set of motivators—time pressure, availability, and temptation—apply at work.

Another key concept in health behavior is the idea of self-efficacy. Simplistically stated, self-efficacy is the confidence people have in their own ability to accomplish a given goal. Many people are familiar with the concept of the self-fulfilling prophesy. When people believe they are doomed to failure, they probably are—not due to the hand of fate, but because of their own lack of confidence. The concept of self-efficacy is applied regularly by many top professional athletes when they use techniques like visualization to work on their "inner game." By visualizing themselves winning their events, these athletes are increasing their self-efficacy.

Another important concept is that changing behavior is not an event but, rather, a process. Let us consider Jim's attempts to stop smoking cigarettes. Over the years he has tried to quit several times but each time he started smoking again sooner or later. Clearly, Jim understands the health hazards of smoking. Before he starts another attempt to quit, he makes sure he is ready by psyching himself up. Then he dives in, sometimes trying nicotine replacement patches to help him get through the nicotine withdrawal. But he always goes back to cigarettes. So what is missing?

Quitting smoking is a process that begins with the realization that smoking is creating problems. Once Jim realizes that quitting is something he should seriously consider, he needs to weigh the positives of smoking (Jim uses cigarettes to manage stress and takes pleasure from smoking) against the negatives (health risks) to see if he is ready to give quitting a try. Even though Jim believed during previous attempts that he was prepared because he had steeled himself for the challenges of quitting, he hadn't really thought through all of the reasons why he wanted to quit so he could use them to stay motivated when his will flagged.

Jim's next step is getting prepared to quit by making a specific plan for how his attempt will fit in with his usual activities and then contingency plans for coping with temptation. Jim thought he was prepared in the past, but was he really? Jim didn't have a plan for handling the urge created by situations when he usually smoked, like with his morning coffee or when he smelled the smoke of other people's cigarettes. Because Jim didn't know what to do if he slipped and had a cigarette, one cigarette meant a failed attempt to quit.

The next step in the process would be actually trying to quit—the event. Yet even the event of quitting is really a process—after how long can someone be said to have quit? A day? A week? A month? A lifetime? Staying quit, or retaining any behavior over the long term has two parts—the action of initiating the behavior and then maintaining the behavior.

Finally, changing behavior is not solely an internal process. Behavior change is done in the context of people's environment. External influences include

- *Social mores.* For example, in some social circles smoking cigarettes is frowned on; in others it is considered "cool."

- *Accepted norms of behavior.* Is it acceptable to disregard physician instructions, or does a patient believe that a doctor's advice should be adhered to strictly?

• *Interaction with the environment.* Do the person's interactions with the environment support or defeat the
change in behavior? Is Jim living with someone who
loves to bake or with another smoker?

Part One of this book explores these concepts and the leading
models of behavior change.

Application of Behavioral Science
to Change Health Behavior

Simply using models to understand health behavior is not the
goal—it is to apply that understanding to the development of more
effective behavior change tools, interventions, and programs. Let
us look at examples of how some of the principles of health behavior change can be used to determine the strategy and content of
interventions designed to change health behavior.

Applying Models to Change Health Behavior

Health behavior is a highly individual issue. Each person has a very
different combination of background, culture, health risks, health
beliefs, motivators, learning style, environment, goals, and expectations. To apply the models effectively requires the ability to indi-
vidualize the program to these characteristics as closely as possible.
Table 1.2 illustrates how one model of health behavior, Bandura's
social cognitive theory, can be applied in the development of
behavior-based health management programs.

In addition to the models of health behavior, an effective intervention program will integrate good instructional design and learning principles and use media that facilitate a high degree of
individualization.

A comparative meta-analysis by Mullen, Green, and Persinger
(1985) of various patient education interventions used in clinical
trials demonstrated that the magnitude of the intervention's effect

Table 1.2.   Applications of Social Cognitive Theory.

Concept	Definition	Implications and Uses
Environment	Factors external to the person	Develop social support
Situation	Person's perception of environment	Correct misperceptions and promote healthful norms
Behavioral capability	Knowledge and skill	Promote learning and provide skills training
Expectations	Anticipatory outcomes	Model positive outcomes of behavior
Expectancies	Value person places on outcome	Present outcomes of change that have functional meaning
Self-control	Personal regulation of goal-directed behavior	Provide opportunities for self-monitoring, goal setting, problem solving, and self-rewards
Observational learning	Modeling behavior from watching actions and outcomes of others	Include credible role models of targeted behavior
Reinforcements	Responses to behavior that change likelihood of recurrence	Promote self-initiated rewards and incentives
Self-efficacy	Person's confidence in performing a behavior	Approach behavioral change in small, specific steps to ensure success
Emotional coping responses	Strategies or tactics to deal with emotional stimuli	Provide training in problem solving and stress management
Reciprocal determinism	Interaction between person, behavior, and environment	Consider multiple avenues to behavioral change

on knowledge and behavior could be predicted based on a quality rating of the intervention's application of several principles of education: consonance, relevance, individualization, feedback, reinforcement, and facilitation.

Because the effect of an intervention on patient knowledge and behavior directly correlates with the rating, it naturally follows that applying the educational principles included as part of the rating scale enables the developer of a patient education program to create an effective intervention. In a 1995 publication, I suggested methods for applying these criteria to the development of effective patient education interventions (Toscani and Patterson, 1995, pp. 36–39, 44). Table 1.3 summarizes those recommendations.

Furthermore, Mullen, Green, and Persinger (1985) showed that combinations of methods were more effective than single methods because combinations provide patients with the opportunity for multiple learning experiences. The use of multiple methods is also more likely to accommodate individual learning abilities or preferences.

Part Two of this book discusses the development of behavioral health programs.

Implementing Behavior Change in Health and Disease Management Programs

There are a number of ways behavior change components can be delivered in health and disease management programs. Because of the need for a high degree of individualization for effective behavior change, many successful programs have depended on interpersonal interaction. This interaction is often delivered in a one-to-one setting by specialized educators or case managers. Group interactions are also frequently used because they have the added benefit of enabling people who have concerns in common to share their experiences. These methods have the disadvantages of being resource intensive, being restricted in the number of people that can be reached practically, and possibly presenting logistical barriers

Table 1.3.   Applications of Educational Principles to Program Design.

Criteria	Description	Example
Consonance	Degree of fit between program and its objectives, or degree to which communication is directed toward accomplishing the intended outcome	In intervention to improve proper bronchodilator usage, teaching benefits of inhaler without showing how to use it would be insufficient.
Relevance	Degree to which intervention is geared to patient, including reading level and visual acuity	Program should be tailored to patient's knowledge, beliefs, circumstances, and prior experience, determined by pretests, baseline questionnaires, or interviews.
Individualization	Allows patients to have personal questions answered or instructions paced according to individual learning progress	Because patients learn in different ways and at different rates, a program is more likely to be effective if the education is tailored to individual needs.
Feedback	Helps patients learn by providing a measuring stick to determine how much progress they are making, if any	Feedback can be based on achieved learning objectives (such as increased knowledge about a given subject) or outcomes (such as increased adherence to a medication regimen).

Table 1.3.   (continued)

Criteria	Description	Example
Reinforcement	Components of the program (other than feedback) designed to reward the desired behavior	Praise and congratulations are very effective in rewarding changed behavior.
Facilitation	Measures taken to accomplish desired actions or eliminate obstacles	For example, a seven-day pill box facilitates patient's ability to adhere to medication schedule or free medication eliminates obstacle of cost.

to some of the people who would benefit most from participation. Programs such as Weight Watchers, Smokenders, and the Arthritis Self-Management Program (a self-care education program administered by the Arthritis Foundation) would fall into this category.

With advances in database-driven communications and information technology over the past decade, highly individualized education, skill development, and behavior change programs can be delivered much more cost effectively. Call centers staffed with counselors, both clinical professionals and laypeople, using databases of patient information and computer-driven best practice algorithms can deliver highly effective behavior change programs. One example of such a program is the Free and Clear smoking cessation program, developed and implemented by Group Health Cooperative Puget Sound. Another new technology—database-driven tailored demand publishing—has been shown to be significantly more effective in changing behavior than standard printed materials (Campbell and others, 1994; Skinner, Strecher, and Hospers, 1994, pp. 12–13; Strecher and others, 1994, pp. 290–291).

However, although these technologies have the benefits of lower cost and broad distribution, they do not have the same impact as interpersonal interactions.

Video has been shown to be a medium with a potential impact equal to group interactions (Meyers, Barclay, Whelan, and Graves, 1996). Highly individualized multimedia applications are now being developed to capitalize on the rapid advances and growth of the Internet and the convergence of computers and broadband technology. These applications hold the promise of further reducing distribution costs, improving access, and increasing impact to a level approaching interpersonal interactions.

Part Three of this book discusses current and future delivery of behavior change programs.

Measurement and Interpretation of Intervention Results

One of the fundamental questions that must be asked about any intervention is: How do I know how well it worked or if it worked at all? When this question is posed about a clinical intervention like a medication, device, or procedure, there is often a relatively straightforward answer. A well-designed controlled trial of an antihypertensive medication will demonstrate clearly whether the medication does or does not lower blood pressure and, following that trial, whether the medication lowers the blood pressure of an individual patient. Because behavioral programs do not have direct physiological effects, there are differences in both what is measured and how the measurements are made. In addition, because behavioral interventions are often designed to improve more subjective types of outcomes, such as quality of life and satisfaction, different measurement approaches are required, as outlined in Table 1.4.

Part Four of this book discusses measurement techniques and selection of appropriate end points.

Table 1.4. **Examples of Measurable End Points in Behavioral Programs.**

Outcomes	End Points
Clinical outcomes	• Early recognition of deterioration in condition • Tolerance of side effects • Adherence to medication regimen • Adherence to follow-up care • Adherence to lifestyle recommendations
Health-related quality of life	• Physical function • Emotional function • Social function
Patient satisfaction	• Quality of physician-patient interaction • Self-efficacy
Utilization	• Direct —Use of emergency services —Inpatient hospital admissions —Physician visits —Medication • Indirect —Absenteeism —Productivity

What to Expect from This Book

The objective of this book is to provide a sound, focused explanation of behavior change theory to establish a foundation for integrating health behavior change into health and disease management programs. After reading this book, you can expect to

• Understand the importance of integrating a patient-centric approach into health and disease management programs

- Understand the theoretical basis for health-related behavior change and the evidence that supports these theories

- Be able to apply behavioral theory in development of health behavior change interventions

- Be familiar with the range of possible intervention methods and their relative advantages and disadvantages in developing behavior change interventions

- Have a working knowledge of the issues involved in measuring, interpreting, and applying results

References

The Boston Consulting Group. *The Promise of Disease Management*. Boston: The Boston Consulting Group, 1995.

Campbell, M. K., and others. "Improving Dietary Behavior: The Effectiveness of Tailored Messages in Primary Care Settings." *American Journal of Public Health*, 1994, 84, 783–787.

Department of Health and Human Services. *Smoking Cessation*. Clinical Practice Guideline no. 18. Centers for Disease Control and Prevention, Agency for Health Care Policy and Research. Atlanta: Department of Health and Human Services, 1996.

"The Disease Management Strategic Research Study and Resource Guide." National Managed Health Care Congress, 1988.

Ellrodt, G., and others. "Evidence-Based Disease Management." *JAMA: Journal of the American Medical Association*, 1997, 278, 1687–1692.

Meyers, A. W., Barclay, D. R., Whelan, J. P., and Graves, T. J. "An Evaluation of a Television-Delivered Behavioral Weight Loss Program: Are the Ratings Acceptable?" *Journal of Consulting and Clinical Psychology*, Feb. 1996, 64(1), 172–178.

Medstat Group, Ann Arbor, Mich. Reported in *Reuters News*, Aug. 25, 1999.

Mullen, P. D., Green, L. W., and Persinger, G. S. "Clinical Trials of Patient Education for Chronic Conditions: A Comparative Meta-analysis of Intervention Types." *Preventive Medicine*, 1985, 14, 753–781.

Musich, S. A., Burton, W. N., and Edington, D. W. "Costs and Benefits of Prevention and Disease Management." *Disease Management Health Outcomes*, 1999, 5(3), 153–166.

Peterson, C. "A Team Approach to Chronic Care." *HMO Magazine*, 1995, 36, 39.

Prochaska, J. O., Redding, C. A., and Evers, K. "The Transtheoretical Model and Stages of Change." In K. Glanz, F. M. Lewis, and B. K. Rimer (eds.), *Health Behavior and Health Education: Theory, Research, and Practice*. (2nd ed.) San Francisco: Jossey-Bass, 1997.

Skinner, C. S., Strecher, V. J., and Hospers, H. "Physicians' Recommendations for Mammography: Do Tailored Messages Make a Difference?" *American Journal of Public Health*, Jan. 1994, 84(1).

Strecher, V. J., and others. "The Effects of Computer-Tailored Smoking Cessation Messages in Family Practice Settings." *Journal of Family Practice*, 1994, 39(3).

Toscani, M. R., and Patterson, R. B. "Evaluating and Creating Effective Patient Education Programs." *Drug Benefit Trends*, 1995, 7(9).

The Vanderveer Group, Fort Washington, Penn. "Understanding the Physician Audience for a Hypertension Wellness Plan." Sept. 1991.

Part I

. . . .

The Role of Patient Behavior
in Health and Disease Management

In their frailties, motivations, intentions, and capacity to change, patients with chronic diseases and conditions are merely human. The profound difference for these patients is the amplified impact of human foibles and unhealthy behavior on their life and health. The benefits of health and disease management ultimately hinge on the patient's sustained participation in a carefully organized regimen of prevention, treatments, therapies, and self-management. Patient noncompliance with the prescribed course will unravel the best-laid plans of program architects.

To improve outcomes in health and disease management, one must first ask what makes patients sometimes act contrary to their own best interests. Even seasoned clinicians too often misunderstand why otherwise reasonable patients may fail to follow the simplest instructions and heed sound medical advice. Because health care providers have struggled for so long with this issue, common myths about health-related behavior abound. Clinicians are sometimes defeated by a fear of powerlessness ("Nothing I do will change this patient's behavior") or an authoritarian approach ("Of course the patient will do precisely what I tell her to do").

Armed with a deeper knowledge and understanding of health behavior, providers can be much more effective in influencing patients toward full compliance and participation in their plan of care.

In Part One we present an overview of health and disease management from the patient's perspective. Our discussion touches on the prevailing theoretical models as well as practical ways to change patient behavior.

In Chapter Two, Karen Glanz and Brian Oldenburg survey the common ground on which current theories and models rest. Taking the patient's point of view, they focus on core beliefs, perceptions, and attitudes behind various health-related behavior. Central to their discussion are the formidable barriers along every patient's journey: finding the motivation to change, declaring the intention to change, and taking the actions necessary to accomplish a lasting change in health behavior.

Chapter Three enumerates the dominant theoretical models that academicians use to explain health-related behavior. Celeste Cafiero and Fern Carness explain how to choose and apply these theoretical models in determining the content and approach of any intervention whose goal is to change or influence health-related behavior.

Subsequent parts of the book build on the theories and models introduced in these first two chapters. As researchers have developed these powerful new ways of understanding patient behavior, health and disease managers have incorporated them in new program designs and implementation strategies. More and more have managed to effect significant changes in patient behavior as well as measurable improvements in interventions and outcomes based on this firm foundation of scientific investigation and disciplined thought.

Utilizing Theories and Constructs Across Models of Behavior Change

Karen Glanz, Brian Oldenburg

Neville is an active, energetic forty-nine-year-old professor who was a competitive cyclist in his twenties and thirties. His demanding work has taken its toll on his health habits recently. He has taken up smoking, rarely exercises, and often overeats. Following a heart attack, he is very anxious to resume his busy schedule and still thinks of himself as the young athlete with boundless energy and ambition. Could this attitude affect his adherence to a cardiac rehabilitation regimen? Will medical restrictions on his diet and activity make him feel depressed, fatalistic, and unmotivated?

Health professionals who work with medical and surgical patients and provide them with advice on health and lifestyle are often disappointed with their poor adherence to treatment even in response to relatively simple medical prescriptions. Poor adherence often arises because patients do not have the necessary behavioral skills to make the prescribed changes or they might not understand the importance of such changes and may even believe that they pose an additional risk to their health. Or a patient might be experiencing an emotional dysfunction like depression or anxiety that will be a major barrier to compliance.

Traditionally it has been assumed that the relationship between knowledge, attitudes, and behavior is a simple and direct one. Indeed, over the years many health education programs have been based on the premise that if people understand the health conse-quences of a particular behavior, they will modify it accordingly. Moreover, the argument goes, if people have a negative attitude toward an existing lifestyle practice and a positive attitude toward change, they will make healthful changes. However, we now know from research conducted over the past thirty years that the rela-tionships between knowledge, awareness of the need to change, intention to change, and an actual change in behavior are very complex indeed.

The Patient's View of the World

Gochman (1988, p. 3) has defined health behavior as "personal attributes such as beliefs, expectations, motives, values, perceptions, and other cognitive elements; personality characteristics, including affective and emotional states and traits; and overt behavior pat-terns, actions and habits that relate to health maintenance, health restoration and health improvement."

This definition of health behavior not only implies a complex set of interrelationships between perceptions, cognitions, emotions, and habits, but also recognizes that these personal attributes are influenced by, and otherwise reflect, family, social, societal, institu-tional, and cultural determinants.

Chapter Two introduces several models and theories of behav-ior change. Patient educators are fortunate to have so many mod-els from which to choose but may find it challenging to sort out the key issues in various models. In this chapter we focus on important principles and constructs across models. The first principle, illus-trated by Neville's situation described above, is that successful patient education depends on a sound understanding of the patient's view of the world.

Ideally, each patient should be treated as an individual with unique circumstances and health history. Still, epidemiological research indicates that certain demographic subgroups differ in terms of risk factors and health behavior. Understanding these population trends can help prepare a provider to work with various types of patients. For example, younger persons may feel invulnerable to coronary events and older adults may be managing multiple chronic conditions. An active middle-aged professional (such as Neville) may place returning to his previous level of activity above important health precautions. These are just a few examples of how population subgroups may differ, serving as a reminder to be sensitive not only to individual circumstances but to group patterns as well (being careful to avoid stereotyping).

Within this general context, various theories and models can guide the search for effective ways to reach and positively motivate patients.

Explanatory Models and Change Models

Cynthia suffers from asthma and finds it difficult to control while she cares for her two school-age children and works part time as a waitress in a small bar-restaurant. She sometimes forgets to take her inhaler with her, often ignores early warning signs of an asthma attack, and finds that her condition is aggravated by the smoke at her workplace.

Theories can guide the search to understand why people do or do not follow medical advice, help identify what information is needed to design an effective intervention strategy, and provide insight into how to design a successful educational program (Glanz and Rimer, 1995). Thus, theories and models help explain behavior as well as suggest how to develop more effective ways to influence and change behavior. These types of theory often have different emphases but are quite complementary (Glanz, Lewis, and Rimer, 1997). For Cynthia, understanding why her asthma flares up is a step toward successful management, but even the best explanations won't be enough by themselves to fully guide change to improve her health and reduce suffering. Some type of change model will also be needed.

Multiple Levels of Influence

Many social, cultural, and economic factors contribute to the development, maintenance, and change of health behavior patterns. Physiological and psychological factors, acquired habits, and knowledge about preventive or risk-reducing behavior are important individual determinants of health-related behavior. Families, social relationships, socioeconomic status, and culture are also important influences.

For health education interventions to be effective, they must be targeted not only at individuals but also at the interpersonal, organizational, and community factors that affect choices about health behavior (Glanz and Rimer, 1995; Oldenburg, 1992; Stokols, 1992). This is clearly illustrated when one thinks of the context of Cynthia's attempts to control her asthma: she is busy caring for her children, works in a smoky environment, and has many demands on her other than self-care. Her behavioral choices are in fact quite complex and clearly determined not only by multiple factors but also by factors at multiple levels.

Traditionally, patient educators have focused on intraindividual factors such as a person's beliefs, knowledge, and skills. Contemporary thinking (and an analysis of Cynthia's scenario) suggests that thinking beyond the individual to the social milieu and environment can enhance the chance of successful health promotion and patient education. Health providers can and should work toward understanding the various levels of influence that affect the patient's behavior and health status.

Definitions and Distinctions

A theory is a set of interrelated concepts, definitions, and propositions that presents a systematic view of events or situations by specifying relations among variables in order to explain and predict the events or situations. The notion of generality or broad application is important, as is testability (van Ryn and Heaney, 1992).

Even though various theoretical models of health behavior may reflect the same general ideas (Cummings, Becker, and Maile, 1980; Weinstein, 1993), each theory employs a unique vocabulary to articulate the specific factors considered to be important. Theories vary in the extent to which they have been conceptually developed and empirically tested.

Health behavior and the guiding concepts for influencing it are too complex to be explained by a single unified theory. Models draw on a number of theories to help understand a specific problem in a particular setting or context. They are often informed by more than one theory as well as by empirical findings. The PRECEDE-PROCEED model by Green and Kreuter (1991), social marketing, and ecological planning approaches are models that support program planning processes and are widely used in health promotion and education (Glanz and Rimer, 1995; Glanz, Lewis, and Rimer, 1997).

Concepts are the major components of a theory; they are the building blocks or primary elements. Concepts can vary in the extent to which they have meaning or can be understood outside the context of a specific theory. When concepts are developed or adopted for use in a particular theory they are called constructs. Variables are the empirical counterparts or operational forms of constructs (Green and Lewis, 1986). They specify how a construct is to be measured in a specific situation. It is important to keep in mind that variables should be matched to constructs when identifying what should be assessed in the evaluation of a theory-driven program.

Behavior Change As a Process

Emma is thirty-five pounds overweight and was recently diagnosed with high blood cholesterol. Her doctor has given her a strict low-fat, low-calorie diet and stressed the importance of losing weight to reduce her cholesterol and risk of heart disease. She looks over the diet instructions and feels overwhelmed—it's so different from how she eats now, she doesn't think she can follow it.

Sustained behavior change involves multiple actions and adaptations over time. Some people may not be ready to attempt changes, some may be thinking about attempting change, and others may have already begun implementing behavioral modifications. One central issue that has gained wide acceptance in recent years is the simple notion that behavior change is a process, not an event. It is important to think of the change process as one that occurs in stages. It is not a question of someone deciding one day to stop smoking and the next day becoming an ex-smoker. Likewise, Emma won't be able to dramatically change her eating pattern all at once. The idea that behavior change occurs in a number of steps is not particularly new, but it has gained wider recognition in the past few years. Indeed, various multistage theories of behavior change date back more than fifty years to the work of Lewin (1935), McGuire (1984), Weinstein (1993), Marlatt and Gordon (1985), and others (Glanz, Lewis, and Rimer, 1997).

The notion of readiness to change, or stage of change, has been examined in health behavior research and found useful in explaining and predicting a variety of behavior. Prochaska, Velicer, DiClemente, and their colleagues have been leaders in beginning to formally identify the dynamics and structure of change that underlie both self-mediated and clinically-facilitated health behavior change. The construct of *stage of change* is a key element of their transtheoretical model of behavior change (TTM), which proposes that people are at different stages of readiness to adopt healthful behavior (Prochaska, DiClemente, and Norcross, 1992; Prochaska, Redding, and Evers, 1997).

The five basic stages of change that have been identified include

1. Precontemplation (unaware, not interested in change)
2. Contemplation (thinking about change in the near future)
3. Preparation (making plans to change)
4. Action (actively modifying behavior or environment)
5. Maintenance (continuation of new, healthier behavior)

TTM is considered circular rather than linear, with people entering or exiting at any point. At least for some behavior, such as smoking, it seems to apply equally well to people who self-initiate change and to those who are responding to advice from health professionals.

Although the stages-of-change construct cuts across various circumstances of individuals who need to change or want to change, other theories also address the process of behavior change. Here we look across various models to illustrate four key concerns:

- Motivation versus intention

- Intention versus action

- Changing behavior versus maintaining behavior change

- Biobehavioral factors

Motivation Versus Intention

Emma really wants to lower her cholesterol level but is overwhelmed right now. She needs to care for her sick elderly parents and get her leaky roof fixed before she can concentrate on her own health.

Behavior change is challenging for most people even if they are highly motivated to change. As has already been noted in this chapter, the set of relationships between knowledge, awareness of the need to change, intention to change, and an actual change in behavior are very complex indeed. For individuals who are coping with disease and illness and who are often having to make very significant changes to their lifestyle and other aspects of their lives, this challenge is even greater. According to the transtheoretical model, people in precontemplation are neither motivated nor planning to change, those in contemplation intend to change, and those in preparation are acting on their intentions by taking specific steps toward the action of change (Prochaska, Redding, and Evers, 1997).

The theory of reasoned action (TRA), or theory of planned behavior (TPB)—a more recent version of TRA—was developed by Ajzen and Fishbein (1980) to understand changes in behavior. Fishbein and his associates argue strongly that behavioral intention, rather than generalized attitudes, is the most proximal determinant of behavior (Montaño, Kasprzyk, and Taplin, 1997). In turn, behavioral intentions are influenced by individuals' attitudes about this behavior as well as by their beliefs about what other people think they should do. More recently, perceived behavioral control—a concept closely related to self-efficacy—has been introduced into the TPB as a third, key influence on behavioral intentions. Control beliefs and self-efficacy are discussed in more detail later in the chapter.

Intention Versus Action

The TPB stops short of attempting to predict action per se (Ajzen and Fishbein, 1980; Montaño, Kasprzyk, and Taplin, 1997), whereas the transtheoretical model makes a clear distinction between the stages of contemplation and preparation and overt action (Prochaska, DiClemente, and Norcross, 1992; Prochaska, Redding, and Evers, 1997). A further application of this distinction comes from one of the most researched models of the relationship between cognitive-attitudinal factors and health behavior change, the health belief model (HBM). The HBM proposes that three constellations of factors or determinants are associated with the likelihood of change at the individual level: socioenvironmental and demographic factors, the individual's perception of the threat of disease, and the individual's perception of the potential value of treatment (Strecher and Rosenstock, 1997, pp. 41–59). If all these factors point in the direction of favorably perceiving change, a person is considered predisposed to action, or intending to act. It is only when a cue to action sets a further process in motion that he or she actually moves into action.

Changing Behavior Versus Maintaining Behavior Change

Neville quit smoking while in the hospital after his heart attack, but he couldn't resist the urge to start smoking again during his next visit to his in-laws.

Even where there is good initial compliance to a lifestyle change program (for example, quitting smoking, changing diet, or increasing physical activity), relapse is very common. Up to 80 percent of smokers who quit smoking relapse within twelve months. Many overweight persons are able to lose weight only to regain it within a year. Thus, it has become clear to researchers and clinicians that undertaking initial behavior changes and maintaining behavior change require different types of strategies. The transtheoretical model distinction between action and maintenance stages implicitly addresses this phenomenon (Prochaska, DiClemente, and Norcross, 1992; Prochaska, Redding, and Evers, 1997). The relapse prevention model of Marlatt and Gordon (1985) specifically focuses on strategies for dealing with maintenance of a recently changed behavior. It involves developing self-management and coping strategies and establishing new behavior patterns that emphasize perceived control, environmental management, and improved self-efficacy—an eclectic mix drawn from social cognitive theory (SCT) (Bandura, 1986), theory of planned behavior (Montaño, Kasprzyk, and Taplin, 1997), applied behavioral analysis, and the forerunners of the stages-of-change model (Weinstein, 1993; Green and Lewis, 1986; Lewin, 1935; McGuire, 1984).

Biobehavioral Factors

The theories described thus far have some important limitations, many of which are only now beginning to be understood. Notably, in addictive or addiction-like behavior there are other important determinants of behavior that may be physiological or metabolic or both. Among the best known are the addictive effects of nicotine, alcohol, and some drugs. Physiological factors increase psychological cravings and create withdrawal syndromes that may impede even highly motivated persons from changing their behavior. There is also mounting evidence that genetic predispositions vary and may make some people more prone to certain addictions than others. Some behavior changes (for example, weight loss) also affect energy metabolism and make long-term risk factor reduction an even greater challenge than it would be if it depended on cognitive-behavioral factors alone. These biobehavioral resistances to change can be modified in part by pharmacological solutions (such as nicotine replacement therapy), but research now suggests that these aids are ineffective unless they are complemented by rigorous efforts at behavior modification.

Barriers to Actions and Decisional Balance

Cynthia knows that she is exposed to smoke at work and is struggling to come up with a way to control her asthma without sacrificing her job.

Cynthia's need to support herself and her family constitutes an obstacle, or barrier, to healthful action. According to social cognitive theory (one of the most widely used theories in health psychology, health education, and public health and an updated version of social learning theory), a central determinant of behavior involves the interaction between individuals and their environment (Bandura, 1986). Behavior and environment are said to continuously interact and influence one another, which is known as the principle of reciprocal determinism.

The concept of barriers to action, or perceived barriers, can be found in several theories of health behavior either explicitly or as an application. It is part of social cognitive theory, the health belief model, and the PRECEDE-PROCEED model. An extension of the concept of barriers to action involves the net benefits of action, also referred to as the *benefits minus barriers* in the health belief model.

In the transtheoretical model, there are parallel constructs labelled as the *pros* (the benefits of change) and *cons* (the costs of change). Taken together, these constructs are known as *decisional balance*, or the pros minus cons, similar to the net benefits of action in the health belief model.

The idea that individuals engage in weighing the relative pros and cons of actions has its origins in Janis and Mann's model of decision making (1977), published more than twenty years ago in their seminal book *Decision Making: A Psychological Analysis of Conflict*, although the idea had emerged much earlier in social psychological discourse. Lewin's (1935) idea of force field analysis, the health belief model's exposition of psychological risk-benefit analysis, and other work on persuasion and decision counseling by Janis and Mann pre-dated that important work. Indeed, this notion is basic to models of rational decision making, in which people intellectually think about the advantages and disadvantages, obstacles and facilitators, barriers and benefits, and pros and cons of engaging in a particular action.

Control Beliefs and Self-Efficacy

Emma knows that she should not only follow a healthy diet but also begin to exercise more regularly. She doesn't feel very much in control of her free time because of her elderly parents' needs. And she has never been athletic, so her self-confidence about being able to exercise consistently is low.

Emma's control beliefs and self-efficacy are holding her back from achieving better health. These deterrents to change are common and can be found in several models of health behavior, including social cognitive theory, the health belief model, the theory of planned behavior, and the relapse prevention model. One of the most important challenges for these models—and ultimately for health professionals who apply them—is to enhance perceived behavioral control and increase self-efficacy, thereby improving patients' motivation and persistence in the face of obstacles.

Social cognitive theory explains human behavior in terms of a three-way, dynamic, reciprocal model in which personal factors, environmental influences, and behavior continually interact. SCT synthesizes concepts and processes from cognitive, behavioristic, and emotional models of behavior change so it can be readily applied to a variety of patient education situations. A basic premise of SCT is that people learn not only through their own experiences but also by observing the actions of others and the results of those actions. Key constructs of social cognitive theory that are relevant to nutritional intervention include observational learning, reinforcement, self-control, and self-efficacy (Glanz and Rimer, 1995; Glanz and Eriksen, 1993; Bandura, 1986). Principles of behavior modification, which have often been used to promote behavioral change, are derived from SCT. Some elements of patient education interventions based on SCT constructs of self-control, reinforcement, and self-efficacy include goal-setting, self-monitoring, and behavioral contracting (Glanz and Eriksen, 1993).

Self-efficacy, or a person's confidence in his or her ability to take action and to persist in that action despite obstacles or challenges, seems to be especially important for influencing health behavior and dietary change efforts (Bandura, 1997). The leading articulators of the health belief model have also recommended that the construct of self-efficacy be included in the HBM when it is applied to lifestyle behavior change (Rosenstock, Strecher, and Becker, 1988). Perceived behavioral control, a construct that was explicitly added to the theory of planned behavior recently, is closely related to self-efficacy. However, in TPB, it is more specific in its premise that individuals hold beliefs about how well they can persist in the face of specific obstacles or facilitating conditions (Montaño, Kasprzyk, and Taplin, 1997).

Health providers can make deliberate efforts to increase patients' self-efficacy using three types of strategies:

1. Setting small, incremental, and achievable goals

2. Using formalized behavioral contracting to establish goals and specify rewards

3. Monitoring and reinforcing the behavior change, including patient self-monitoring by record keeping (Glanz and Rimer, 1995)

Selecting or Constructing a Model with "Good Fit"

Effective patient education depends on marshaling the most appropriate theory and practice strategies for a given situation (Glanz and Rimer, 1995). Some theories will be better suited than others for particular individuals and situations. For example, when attempting to overcome women's personal barriers to obtaining mammograms, the health belief model may be useful. The transtheoretical model may be especially useful in developing smoking cessation interventions. When trying to change physicians' patient counseling practices by instituting reminder systems, the PRECEDE-PROCEED model may be most suitable. The choice of the most fitting theory or theories should begin with identifying the problem, goal, and units of practice, not with simply selecting a theoretical framework because it is intriguing or familiar.

When it comes to practical application, theories are often judged in the context of activities of fellow practitioners. To apply the criterion of usefulness to a theory, most providers are concerned with whether it is consistent with everyday observations (Glanz and Rimer, 1995). In contrast, researchers usually make scientific judgments of how well a theory conforms to observable reality when empirically tested. Therefore, patient educators should review the research literature periodically to supplement their first-hand experience and that of their colleagues.

A central premise in applying to patient education an understanding of the influences on health behavior is that you can gain an understanding of a patient through an interview or written assessment. In this way you can focus in on that individual's readiness for change, self-efficacy, knowledge level, and so on. Clearly, it is necessary to select a short list of factors to evaluate, which may differ depending on clinical risk factors or a patient's history. Once there is a good understanding of a person's cognitive and behavioral situation, the intervention can be personalized, or tailored. Tailored messages and feedback have been found to be promising strategies for encouraging healthful behavior changes in primary care, community, and home-based settings (Campbell and others, 1994; Beresford and others, 1997; Brug and others, 1998).

Practitioners of health promotion and education both benefit from and are challenged by the eclectic nature of their endeavor. For the unprepared, the choices can be overwhelming; but for those who understand the commonalities and differences among theories of health behavior and health education, the growing knowledge base can provide a firm foundation on which to build. Theories and models are useful because they enrich, inform, and complement the practical technologies of health promotion and education.

Conclusion

Many challenges remain for developing practical and effective patient education interventions that can be adopted in health care practice. The accumulated knowledge suggests that frequent patient monitoring, reminders, family involvement, and group support are likely to help improve adherence. Further, research to date indicates that successful interventions with patients should include baseline assessment, individualized dietary recommendations, goal setting, assessing stage of change, self-monitoring, and self-management strategies for maintaining behavior change (Van Horn and Kavey, 1997). Motivating and guiding adult patients to change remains a multidisciplinary challenge, a health care goal, and an important public health challenge for the twenty-first century.

References

Ajzen, I., and Fishbein, M. *Understanding Attitudes and Predicting Social Behavior.* Englewood Cliffs, N.J.: Prentice-Hall, 1980.

Bandura, A. *Self-efficacy: The Exercise of Control.* New York: Freeman, 1997.

Bandura, A. *Social Foundations of Thought and Action: A Social Cognitive Theory.* Englewood Cliffs, N.J.: Prentice-Hall, 1986.

Beresford, S. A., and others. "A Dietary Intervention in Primary Care Practice: The Eating Patterns Study." *American Journal of Public Health*, 1997, 87, 610–616.

Brug, J., and others. "The Impact of Computer-Tailored Feedback and Iterative Feedback on Fat, Fruit, and Vegetable Intake." *Health Education and Behavior*, 1998, 25, 517–531.

Campbell, M. K., and others. "Improving Dietary Behavior: The Effectiveness of Tailored Messages in Primary Care Settings." *American Journal of Public Health*, 1994, 84, 783–787.

Cummings, K. M., Becker, M. H., and Maile, M. C. "Bringing the Models Together: An Empirical Approach to Combining Variables Used to Explain Health Actions." *Journal of Behavioral Medicine*, 1980, 3, 123–145.

Glanz, K., and Eriksen, M. P. "Individual and Community Models for Dietary Behavior Change." *Journal of Nutrition Education*, 1993, 25, 80–86.

Glanz, K., Lewis, F. M., and Rimer, B. K. (eds.). *Health Behavior and Health Education: Theory, Research, and Practice.* (2nd ed.) San Francisco: Jossey-Bass, 1997.

Glanz, K., and Rimer, B. K. *Theory at a Glance: A Guide for Health Promotion Practice.* Bethesda, Md.: National Cancer Institute, 1995 (National Institutes of Health publication no. 95-3896).

Gochman, D. F. *Health Behavior: Emerging Research Perspectives.* New York: Plenum, 1988.

Green, L. W., and Kreuter, M. W. *Health Promotion Planning: An Educational and Environmental Approach.* (2nd ed.) Mountain View, Calif.: Mayfield, 1991.

Green, L. W., and Lewis, F. M. *Measurement and Evaluation in Health Education and Health Promotion.* Mountain View, Calif.: Mayfield, 1986.

Janis, I., and Mann, L. *Decision Making: A Psychological Analysis of Conflict.* New York: Free Press, 1977.

Lewin, K. *A Dynamic Theory of Personality.* New York: McGraw-Hill, 1935.

Marlatt, A. G., and Gordon, J. R. *Relapse Prevention: Maintenance Strategies in the Treatment of Addictive Behaviors.* New York: Guilford Press, 1985.

McGuire, W. J. "Public Communication as a Strategy for Inducing Health Promoting Behavioral Change." *Preventive Medicine*, 1984, 13, 299–313.

Montaño, D., Kasprzyk, D., and Taplin, S. H. "The Theory of Reasoned Action and Theory of Planned Behavior." In K. Glanz, F. M. Lewis, and B. K. Rimer (eds.), *Health Behavior and Health Education: Theory, Research, and Practice.* (2nd ed.) San Francisco: Jossey-Bass, 1997, pp. 85–112.

Oldenburg, B. "Lifestyle Change and Cardiovascular Disease: Principles and Practice." *Australian Family Physician*, 1992, 21, 1289–1296.

Prochaska, J. O., DiClemente, C. C., and Norcross, J. C. "In Search of How People Change: Applications to Addictive Behaviors." *American Psychologist*, 1992, 47, 1102–1114.

Prochaska, J. O., Redding, C. A., and Evers, K. "The Transtheoretical Model and Stages of Change." In K. Glanz, F. M. Lewis, and B. K. Rimer (eds.), *Health Behavior and Health Education: Theory, Research, and Practice.* (2nd ed.) San Francisco: Jossey-Bass, 1997.

Rosenstock, I. M., Strecher, V. J., and Becker, M. H. "Social Learning Theory and the Health Belief Model." *Health Education Quarterly*, summer 1988, 15(2), 175–183.

Stokols, D. "Establishing and Maintaining Healthy Environments: Toward a Social Ecology of Health Promotion." *American Psychologist*, 1992, 47, 6–22.

Strecher, V. J., and Rosenstock, I. M. "The Health Belief Model." In K. Glanz, F. M. Lewis, and B. K. Rimer (eds.), *Health Behavior and Health Education: Theory, Research, and Practice.* (2nd ed.) San Francisco: Jossey-Bass, 1997.

Van Horn, L., and Kavey, R. E. "Diet and Cardiovascular Disease Prevention: What Works?" *Annals of Behavioral Medicine*, 1997, 19, 197–212.

van Ryn, M., and Heaney, C. A. "What's the Use of Theory?" *Health Education Quarterly*, 1992, 19, 315–330.

Weinstein, N. D. "Testing Four Competing Theories of Health-Protective Behavior." *Health Psychology*, 1993, 12, 324–333.

· ·

Applying the Theory

Models of Behavior Change

Celeste Cafiero, Fern Carness

Jane feels an icy wave of terror as she finds a stony lump in her breast. When was her last mammogram? What had she read recently on exercise, diet, and breast cancer? Why is she still ten pounds overweight? Jane is an informed, educated woman, yet why has she not changed her behavior to protect her health?

Knowing and doing are very separate variables in the area of health behavior. Didactic information abounds. The large majority of people know basic health recommendations: don't smoke; eat a balanced, low-fat, high-fiber diet; exercise regularly; and take medicine exactly as prescribed (McGinnis, 1993). Yet, by and large, most individuals are failing miserably in their own personal health management. One must ask why. If we know what to do, why we should do it, and how important it is, why do we still fail to change? Applying behavior change theory is one health education strategy for helping to bridge the gap between recommending behavior and helping individuals make the recommended behavior change.

Developing Behavior Change Interventions

Modern health care providers have a much more daunting job than medicine's forefathers. Palliative and restorative remedies of the past did not have a compliance component to grapple with, but today the age of chronic conditions is upon us. Curing and ameliorating chronic diseases require that patients accept self-responsibility for their treatment regimen—both medical and lifestyle. What knowledge and skills can be provided to individuals so that they are able to make a salient contribution to their own personal health management? And what is the best framework for this information for behavior change to be successful both in the short and long term?

Insight into these questions may be found in a comprehensive review of the literature on human behavior change models (Glanz, Lewis, and Rimer, 1997). Why humans do or don't do a specific action is a complex and intriguing topic (explored by Kolb, 1984). In this chapter we will discuss the prevalent models of behavior change and present examples for review that can help in planning the most appropriate disease management programs for a variety of settings. Health behavior is too complex to be explained or influenced by only one intervention model, and no one model has proven to be effective in all situations. Rather, the power of combining several models should be considered for program planning. In the end nothing can replace the power of genuine concern and a caring touch.

Although much of the work on interventions for health behavior change has been conducted during the past few decades, none of this work could have been done without the groundwork laid by theorists early in the century, including Pavlov, Skinner, and Lewin. The timeline shown in Exhibit 3.1 represents some of the historical milestones that have contributed to the growth and application of behavior change theories.

Many examples of the utilization of various behavior change strategies can be found in the work of the U.S. Preventive Services Task Force (1996). Behavior change models have been applied to programs as basic as tuberculosis screening, flu shots, exercise, and nutritional guidelines and as complex as contraception use and HIV prevention. More recently these models have been applied to disease management programs that include both patient compliance

Exhibit 3.1.   Timeline of Health Behavior Models.

1927	Pavlov	
1930s	Skinner	
1935	Lewin	Field Theory and Group Process
1950s	Hochbaum, Rosenstock, Kasl, and Cobb	Health Belief Model (HBM)
1957	Festinger	Cognitive Consistency Model
1958	Heider	Attribution Theory
1968	Slovic and Lichtenstein	Prospect Theory
1972	Sayeki	Multiattribute Utility Theory
1975	Ajzen and Fishbein	Theory of Reasoned Action (TRA)
1975	Rogers	Protection Motivation Theory
1977	Bandura	Social Learning Theory (SLT)
1979	Bettman	Consumer Information Processing Theory
1980	Green	PRECEDE
1982	Kotler	Social Marketing
1982	Leventhal, Zimmerman, and Guttmann	Self-Regulation Theory
1982	Prochaska and DiClemente	Transtheoretical Model
1982	Ajzen	Theory of Planned Behavior (TPB)
1985	Marlatt and Gordon	Relapse Prevention Model (RPM)
1986	Bandura	Social Cognitive Theory (SCT)
1991	Green and Kreuter	PRECEDE-PROCEED
1992	Langer and Warheit	Pre-adult Health Decision-Making Model (PAHDM)

and education components (*Disease State Management Sourcebook*, 1998). Current theories have been used in both client-centered and population-based applications. A blend of components from a variety of successful models have often been combined in an attempt to provoke an individual's "ah ha"—the "teachable moment" that catalyzes behavior change.

As we see in the work done by Kasl and Cobb and others, the average person seeks health information under several circumstances. Reasons for seeking health information vary depending on the behavioral role chosen by the individual, for example:

- Sick role behavior, when restoring health or halting disease is the goal

- Illness behavior, when the identification of appropriate treatment is the reason for action

- Health behavior, when the prevention of illness or early detection is possible (Mechanic, 1983)

But regardless of the model of behavior change at work, the ability of the patient to act on that health information requires self-efficacy and independence, which includes physical and emotional energy often lacking in patients with chronic debilitating conditions. Self-efficacy is a belief in one's ability to make a specific change in a specific situation. Adopting preventive health behavior requires reaching that independent stage where voluntary action is taken to prevent illness and promote health. It is from this point that we can begin to look at the individual models of health behavior change.

It is possible to improve people's health through external controls without changing their behavior—for example, by heart surgery, installing air bags in cars, improving sanitation, or implementing fluoridation. However, in the face of chronic illness, it is ultimately the behavior of the individual that will have the greatest impact on his or her long-term health status. Our review of the various models reveals the recurrent theme of the power of personal health practices.

Health care practitioners who have insight into behavior change models can assist individuals in developing the necessary knowledge, beliefs, and skills to change. And those responsible for designing a program to help manage chronic diseases will need to know which elements of the models have worked in the past, what might work, and what has not worked. Designing effective disease management programs takes more than just putting words on a page, posting on a web site, or dispensing advice by phone. Without a predetermined educational design and structure individuals will not be prepared to use the information they have received.

Behavior change will only last if it is a self-directed process. The self-directed behavior change process has many components, including

- *Self-monitoring.* Observing and becoming aware of one's behavior by charting it creates a benchmark.

- *Goal specification.* Setting short-term goals that are specific, measurable, achievable, and moderately challenging gives objective checkpoints.

- *Stimulus control.* Identifying the cues that trigger the unwanted behavior and developing strategies for dealing with those triggers help patients stay on track.

- *Self-reinforcement.* Rewarding positive behavior regularly with immediate, simple, positive, and tangible rewards improves success.

- *Social support.* Enlisting the help of family, friends, and coworkers increases compliance.

- *Contracting.* Writing down the commitment to personal goals reinforces the behavior.

- *Behavior rehearsal.* Practicing the desired behavior and responses to potential relapse situations helps make the new behavior a habit (Kaplan, Sallis, and Patterson, 1993).

By increasing the number of these self-directed behavior change components included in your program design and encouraging individuals to use as many of these components as possible in their own action plans, you can enhance the likelihood of influencing behavior. Review these features of the components of self-directed behavior change again in more detail before determining a program design:

- *Self-monitoring.* For example, weighing oneself each day or recording each cigarette smoked each day.

  Self-observation of the target behavior increases self-awareness (Watson and Thorpe, 1997).

  Keeping a written record provides a benchmark.

  Reviewing the record provides a basis for defining and measuring the desired behavior.

- *Goal specification.* For example, walking twenty minutes each day to reduce blood pressure to less than 140/90.

  Setting goals that are specific and realistic enhances outcomes.

  Setting goals that are at least moderately challenging leads to higher performance (Strecher, 1995).

  Focusing on the behavior is a means to attaining a health goal.

Setting both short-term and long-term goals increases the likelihood of accomplishment.

• *Stimulus control.* For example, removing the cigarette lighter from the car or laying exercise clothes out the night before.

Identifying the situation (antecedent) that is consistently associated with a behavior and its consequences allows for cue extinction (Watson and Thorpe, 1997).

Inserting a new or alternative cue that triggers the desired behavior increases chances of success.

Increasing awareness of the unconscious component of an unwanted behavior helps diminish its occurrence.

Adapting the physical or social environment to remove temptation encourages compliance (Marlatt and Gordon, 1985).

• *Self-reinforcement.* For example, rewarding oneself with fresh flowers each week for not smoking or using positive self-talk: "I have so much more energy when I've exercised twenty minutes each day."

Determining the "if-then" contingency and reinforcement enhances success.

Using reinforcers that are immediate, simple, tangible, and desirable is best.

Using symbolic reinforcers such as positive self-talk or self-praise is also effective.

Self-reinforcement is more effective than self-punishment.

• *Social support.* For example, asking a friend along on a walk three times a week.

> Social support should come from people you care about and who care about you.
>
> Buddy systems with daily, ongoing contact are most effective.

• *Contracting*

> Writing a contract is a symbolic form of reinforcing commitment to reaching the behavioral goals.
>
> A behavior change contract is specific, measurable, attainable, rewardable, and trackable.

• *Behavior rehearsal.* For example, practicing saying, "No, thank you, I'm full" when someone offers a second portion.

> Regularly modeling or rehearsing the desired behavior increases the likelihood of it becoming the preferred behavior.
>
> Visualizing performing the desired behavior is a powerful form of behavior rehearsal.

Health Belief Model

The health belief model (HBM) came from groundbreaking research in the 1950s done by the U.S. Public Health Service (Mechanic, 1983). Previously, diseases were less curable and medicine was palliative. After World War II the impact of antibiotics and other pharmaceuticals brought the notion of cure and prevention to the forefront (Jones, Jones, and Katz, 1991). Imagine how perplexed health workers must have been at first when people failed to get screened for tuberculosis even though there was now a treatment. Fortunately, researchers at that time were focused on individual variables so they constructed a model that analyzed patients' perceptions of

- Their susceptibility to a disease

- Severity of the disease

- Benefits of treatment or prevention

- Barriers to treatment or prevention

This model hypothesized that individuals will generally not seek treatment or screening unless they have some knowledge of the condition, have some belief of personal vulnerability, and think the condition will be threatening (Ferrini, Edelstein, and Barrett-Connor, 1994). They must have trust in the efficacy of the intervention (perceive a benefit) and have easy access to the process or perceive no insurmountable barriers to their accepting the intervention.

> Phillip has an eighty-six-year-old uncle who has smoked since he was twelve. Although Phillip believes that smoking does cause cancer and that cancer is a condition he wants to avoid, he also believes that he is protected by his genetic makeup. He admits that quitting would be a good thing to do and thinks he can quit whenever he likes. Phillip's lack of belief in his personal susceptibility prevents his taking action on his smoking.

Although the HBM was originally designed as a value-expectancy model to predict the use of a specific preventive health action (Schafer, Keith, and Schafer, 1995), it went through many refinements during the 1970s and 1980s. Investigators including Becker, Maiman, Gochman, and Rosenstock made valuable contributions to the HBM by adding new theoretical elements from more recent models such as reasoned action, social cognitive, and stages of change. By enhancing the HBM in this way a more functional approach for predicting and changing health behavior can be achieved and an applicability to disease management programs can be found (Grodner, 1991).

Within the health belief model, designers of programs need to deal with all of the four elements—susceptibility, severity, benefits, and barriers—to successfully help individuals chart a course for behavior change strategy. Helping individuals address their beliefs about these four elements can improve their receptivity to behavior change and enhance long-term success.

- *Susceptibility*. How ready people are to take a health-related action depends on their perception of their likelihood of susceptibility to that specific illness. Those who believe they are not susceptible or are immune will not take action.

- *Severity*. How serious a person believes the social or physical consequences of the illness are influences their actions. For example, the prospect of facing open heart surgery may convince a person with high cholesterol to begin exercising.

- *Benefits and barriers*. The health recommendation being suggested must be considered feasible and its benefit must outweigh any barriers associated with the action. For example, issues such as cost, access, pain, or fear can keep a person from acting.

Finally, the HBM depends on a cue to action. The cue to action may be internal, such as symptoms of a disease like pain, bleeding, or a lump, or external, such as a physician's recommendation, media campaigns, or community-based program recommendations (Champion, 1997).

Morris had a forty-year-old neighbor who smoked and died from lung cancer. Morris has a young family who keep pestering him to quit smoking. He believes that smoking threatens his health and longevity and would also like to save the money he now spends on cigarettes. Morris feels that he can't stop cold turkey, but he has a friend who was able to stop smoking by attending a local American Lung Association program. The classes are offered at his worksite and he has enrolled for the next program.

With a model as well validated as the HBM, practitioners and program planners have a valuable construct to apply to a practical program design. One example of current use of the HBM can be found in the work of Bond, Aiken, and Somerville (1992). Although the HBM was not originally designed to predict behavior in individuals with a disease, these researchers tested the predictive utility of the HBM for adherence with a diabetic regimen and glycemic control in a chronically ill adolescent population. This study tested the constructs of threat, benefits, and cues in a group of youthful insulin-dependent diabetics. Within the HBM the cue components (internal symptoms such as sweats, nausea and vomiting, and shortness of breath) were found to be most closely associated with adherence. The threat of health consequences for not following the medical regimen were found to actually undermine adherence.

By applying the various components of the HBM to adherence, practitioners and program designers can enhance the effectiveness of behavior change counseling for chronic disease management and improve the outcomes of education and compliance programs.

How can this model be used to help Phillip?

Phillip visits his doctor because he has bronchitis. During the visit his doctor asks if he smokes and Phillip tells him that he does and adds proudly that he has an uncle who is still smoking at age eighty-six.

His doctor shares with him that he can't count on the health history of a relative to protect him from smoking-related disease. His doctor also says that based on Phillip's current bronchitis he may already be experiencing some of the ill effects of his smoking. On the way home, Phillip meets his neighbor, Morris, who has just returned from his stop-smoking class. Phillip thinks, if Morris can do this, so can I!

Theory of Reasoned Action

Bobbie's friends, who are in their mid-forties, were all discussing their mammogram experience over lunch. Bobbie has not yet had a baseline mammogram. Based on the lunch conversation, Bobbie believes that her friends assume that she too has had a mammogram based on her age and risk level. Bobbie makes a note in her calendar to call her doctor for an appointment.

Developed by the social psychologists Ajzen and Fishbein in the 1970s, the theory of reasoned action (TRA) holds that all human behavior is under our own control. The theory asserts that individuals engage in practices that are in their own best self-interest. The TRA predicts behavior based on an individual's intention to perform or not to perform the behavior.

Flo was told by her doctor to take both her blood pressure medications daily. Flo is a bus driver and finds that when she takes her diuretic each morning she needs to urinate frequently. Because this is very inconvenient during her workday, Flo decides that she will only take her "water pill" on her days off but intends to take the other blood pressure pill every day.

Intention is also determined by the individual's attitude about the behavior and what the individual's beliefs are about the subjective norm, that is, what they think other people think about the behavior.

Arty is trying to get his cholesterol level down so he takes his cholesterol-lowering medication every day and plans to exercise three times a week. He believes his wife is worried about his health and she thinks exercise will help him. Arty has signed up for an exercise class at the local YMCA.

Common sense would have us believe that an individual who intends to make a behavior change will do so. Based on TRA, practitioners can influence intention to make a behavior change and increase compliance by influencing the elements of this model. These elements include

- *Behavioral intention.* Will I do or not do the behavior?

- *Attitude toward desired behavior.* Do I think this is a good or bad thing to do?

- *Belief about the behavior.* Do I believe that this behavior will help me reach my goal?

- *Evaluation of consequences.* If I do this behavior will I like the result?

- *Subjective norm.* Do I think others think this is a good or bad thing for me to do?

- *Normative belief.* What do I think others think about this behavior?

- *Motivation or intention to comply.* Do I do what others think I should do? (Hedeker, Flay, and Petraitis, 1996)

How would this model be used to help Flo?

Flo goes back to her doctor for her blood pressure check and finds it has not improved significantly. Flo admits to not taking her diuretic each morning. She is told how important it is for both medications to work together every day and her doctor suggests that she take her diuretic when she gets home from work each day. Once Flo's belief that this medication had to be taken in the morning was corrected, her intention was able to be changed, which influenced her behavior.

Theory of Planned Behavior

The theory of planned behavior (TPB) by Ajzen adds the element of perceived behavioral control to the theory of reasoned action developed by Ajzen and Fishbein described above (Blue, 1995). Perceived behavioral control is how easy or difficult an individual thinks adopting a new behavior will be. Perceived control acknowledges that there is a continuum of control that runs from no control to complete control (Ajzen, 1985).

This model is particularly useful in the area of exercise adherence in which it becomes apparent that social support affects perceived control. In other words, one may feel more control over the behavior when exercising with a friend (Godin and Kok, 1996).

Mara, forty-nine years old, has always wanted to exercise but was never any good at sports in school. Now she feels embarrassed to start so late in life. Her coworker, Thom, is beginning to train for a marathon that happens to fall on Mara's fiftieth birthday next spring. Thom offers to help Mara train in very small, manageable increments (Courneya and McAuley, 1995).

The theory of planned behavior suggests that there are motivational factors influencing how hard one is willing to try to accomplish a goal. The acceptable level of effort is determined by three variables: attitude, subjective norm (as noted in TRA), and perceived control. The TPB asserts that people intend to perform a behavior if they think it is a good thing (evaluate it positively), believe it is important to others (subjective norm), and perceive the behavior to be under their control (perceived control).

First walking for thirty minutes was hard, but Thom showed Mara that she could do it. Soon they were walking each day and then jogging three mornings a week. By the start of spring Mara and Thom had their distance up to eighteen miles and were ready to complete the spring run in celebration of her birthday (Dishman, 1988).

Relapse Prevention Model

It was Jack's best friend's wedding, so what could he do? Daniel, a college roommate, had asked Jack to be his best man. That meant not only attending the wedding reception, but also being responsible for planning a bachelor party. Jack felt planning a wild, alcohol-filled night was expected of him. Jack had just celebrated ninety days of sobriety. The blackouts and the possibility of losing his job had finally taken Jack to a detox program. How could he be best man without drinking?

Dangerous environments and dangerous people are a perfect setup for a relapse for those who are working on a behavior change. In 1985, Marlatt and Gordon proposed a self-management program to support the maintenance phase of a behavior change process. This model focused on teaching individuals how to anticipate and cope with a relapse (Courneya, 1995).

Behavior change programs in the areas of weight loss, smoking cessation, and substance abuse have all experienced high recidivism rates. Making a positive behavior change is merely half the battle; maintaining the new behavior requires knowledge and skill. Furthermore, more than 60 percent of all relapses occur within the first ninety days after initiating a behavior change.

The relapse prevention model takes the position that a lapse or slip is not the same as a relapse. There are two very clear strategies that one can employ to deal with the problem of relapse:

• Avoid the antecedent to a relapse.

• Identify and enhance alternative coping mechanisms.

Once individuals make a behavior change and maintain the new behavior or abstinence, they have a sense of self-efficacy, or perceived control. This sense of control is usually strong until they encounter a high-risk situation. A high-risk situation can be any person, place, or thing that poses a threat to continued progress of the new behavior.

This model suggests that those most likely to relapse are those who exhibit

- Negative emotional states such as anger, depression, or boredom

- Those experiencing interpersonal conflict with friends, coworkers, family members, and others and those exposed to direct or indirect social pressures

To prevent relapse, the individual can avoid high-risk situations by first becoming aware of the trigger and then planning to avoid or escape it or adapt the situation to support the new behavior. In addition, one can plan alternative coping mechanisms that will fend off a lapse (Marlatt and Gordon, 1985). The term *abstinence violation effect* refers to the decrease in self-efficacy that follows a lapse, which can then lead to a relapse (Glasser, 1976). The relapse prevention model teaches that one may circumvent this self-defeating routine by practicing positive thoughts along with avoidance and coping strategies.

> Realizing that the lure of drinking at the bachelor party would be too much for him, Jack agrees to plan the bash but not to attend. He informs Daniel that he will arrange the party but asks other friends in the wedding party to take care of things that evening. In addition, Jack makes a list of alternative coping techniques he can use when the urge to drink hits at the wedding reception. Jack's wife arranges for sparkling apple cider to be available for the champagne toast Jack will give to the newlyweds, thus discouraging a slip or a relapse.

Model of Illness Behavior

> Nanna used to be spry and energetic. At eighty she still cooked for neighbors on special occasions and frequently attended activities in the community center. But lately she was having trouble getting up and out of chairs and bed and felt unsteady when walking. Fearful that this was proof that her health was failing, she withdrew from her activities and became housebound and sedentary.

As our population ages and problems associated with chronic conditions increase, many of the traditional health behavior change models have become inadequate. Often it is our own perception of disability that defines how illness is perceived. In fact, sickness sometimes may be seen as advantageous. As the struggle of living and stress-induced diseases increase, for some people there are alarming advantages to being ill.

The illness literature highlights that patients often see illness differently than the health care provider does (Marlatt and Gordon, 1985). People usually attend to symptoms when they feel discomfort, pain, or a general sense of poor well-being. Yet using sickness (real or imagined) as an excuse to justify release from obligations or as a way to get special attention should not be overlooked (Mechanic, 1995).

> Sara, Nanna's neighbor, sprained her ankle last winter. Her friends began visiting often, bringing her groceries and meals. Sara has refused physical therapy and has not yet returned to her usual activities of daily life.

When planning a behavior intervention, the health care provider needs to assess not only the current condition but the secondary conditions that add to the disability. This includes evaluating the efforts needed to allow participation in health promoting behavior and those that prevent loss of self-efficacy and self-esteem.

As our population ages, more interventions that promote function and independence rather than cure are needed to enhance perceived well-being.

Although there was no pathology in Nanna's case, she became increasingly symptomatic due to her illness perception. The health behavior change necessary here required motivation, coping strategies, and skill training.

> Nanna's doctor recommended physical therapy to improve her strength. The physical therapist was able to alter Nanna's pessimistic self-concept through motivation, teach her useful strategies for coping with her recent weakness, and show her exercises to enhance her strength. With the return of her self-control and an improved sense of well-being, Nanna returned to her daily routines.

What we see here is the impact of subjective health assessment. Much work has been done in the area of predictive tools. It is not quite understood by scientists why it seems that people can assess their own health better than risk factor algorithms or physician assessment can. The major component here seems to be the patient's perception of well-being (Scicchitano and others, 1996).

Because response to symptom management is more important with chronic illness than cure, it becomes apparent that health educators and health care providers can gain great insight by listening to patients' perception of their health status. In addition, practitioners need to be aware of the perceived benefits of being ill that may be barriers to getting well. Help-seeking behavior is initiated differently in "other-defined" versus "self-defined" situations (Schiaffino and Cea, 1995). When health care professionals tell patients that they have a medical condition that needs to be addressed, the patients may not agree or acknowledge the illness themselves. It is easy to see how compliance with a medical regime will differ depending on who defines the need for care. It is with a self-defined illness (patients perceive that they have a medical problem) that we see a greater level of compliance. Helping the patient to understand the condition even in the absence of symptoms can have a striking effect on health behavior and outcomes. Becoming aware of the impact of self-perception of well-being adds another tool to the health care practitioner's tool kit.

Transtheoretical Model—Stages of Change

> Sheila, a stock analyst on Wall Street, walked four extra blocks every day as she went to work to avoid passing the door to the Alcoholics Anonymous meeting hall. Sheila feared that even going near the program would make her think about her drinking. Sheila was not interested in changing her alcohol use; in fact, she refused to discuss her drinking pattern at all.

In a 1980s review of the outcomes of smoking cessation programs, the American Cancer Society found that most smokers quit on their own without any formal intervention (Mechanic, 1983). But the key criterion was that they quit when they were ready. This is important information for all practitioners and program planners because, if people change when they are ready, maybe we can help them get ready.

In the transtheoretical, or stages of change, model, Prochaska and DiClemente propose a circular model of the change process in which the participant can enter or exit at any point (Ferguson, 1987). This model lists the following six stages for overcoming bad habits and forming new health-related behavior:

- *Precontemplation.* People in this stage are not even aware that there is a problem to change. Changing their unhealthy habits is not even on their radar screen. If the topic comes up, they change the subject. Precontemplators avoid information so that they can remain in ignorant bliss. For example, there are scores of smokers who do not believe that smoking is harmful. They stay in denial because it is safe and they fear the unknown circumstances of changing their opinion. The good news is that even precontemplators can change when given the proper tools.

- *Contemplation.* In this stage people may not show it but they are getting ready to make a change. Change is on the horizon. Contemplators truly want to change. They begin to be receptive to information as their awareness increases. In this stage there is also an emotional component that can be evoked by a cue to action, such as a heartfelt public service announcement or a recommendation from a health care provider. This is a good time to have the person specify goals and begin to self-monitor the bad behavior. Contemplators make decisions about changes.

Sheila was surprised when her gynecologist asked her if she smoked and how much she drank as part of her health history during her annual visit. She really hadn't thought about how much she drank each day until then. And it startled her that even though she didn't give a totally honest answer about her daily alcohol consumption, her doctor had suggested she cut back. For the first time Sheila started paying attention to how much she was drinking.

- *Preparation.* Here we find an increased sense of awareness and see that plans are being made to make changes. After making the decision in the contemplation stage, the person in preparation identifies the specific steps that will be taken. The decision to change needs to move up to having the highest priority. Identifying solutions to obstacles and barriers also happens in this preparation stage. It is here that a commitment to the change is forged.

Yes, thought Sheila, if I don't stop drinking I could kill myself—I just missed crashing into that oncoming truck. I may not be so lucky next time. I guess there must be a program in town. I'll call AA and ask about its schedule of meetings.

• *Action*. This stage is when the actual change takes place. Effective change actions require a strong commitment. There are no guarantees, but solid preparation can increase the chance of success. The change process that is helpful here is that of substituting healthy activities for the unwanted behavior. Creating a new healthy habit is sometimes called a positive addiction (Prochaska, Norcross, and DiClemente, 1984).

Sheila stood up. "I'm Sheila, and I am an alcoholic." Joining the AA program was an action she never thought she would take. Yet she now believed she had found the support she needed to stop drinking. Coming to these meetings really helped.

• *Maintenance*. Successful change doesn't end with the action stage (Velicer, Rossi, Prochaska, and DiClemente, 1996). Without a strong plan of action, the newly changed behavior is at risk of relapse. Short-term change programs or easy fixes forget to mention that maintenance is necessary for a lifetime. A plan to avoid slips and lapses is necessary to maintain the new behavior. As Mark Twain said about smoking: "It's easy to quit, I've done it a hundred times."

Thinking things were under control, Sheila felt there was no harm in her having an occasional glass of wine with dinner. However, her maintenance plan reminded her that it was risky. She remembered her friend, Al. He had succumbed to the idea "just one won't hurt" the last time he quit smoking. Now he knew better.

- *Termination*. Finally getting the old behavior completely out of one's life happens in the termination stage. Maintaining the desired behavior is now a natural part of life and does not require constant conscious effort. Although some experts warn never to let one's guard down, there are many kinds of behavior that will fade entirely with time.

It's been twenty years since Al had a cigarette. He never thinks about smoking. Shooting pool surrounded by smokers does not even tempt him. Occasionally he remembers how much he did enjoy smoking, but he also remembers how hard he worked to become a nonsmoker. Al always chooses nonsmoking sections of restaurants and is proud to call himself a nonsmoker.

Social Cognitive Theory

Juan has quit smoking! He knew he could do it and he did. But he can't seem to cut back on his coffee as his cardiologist recommended. Juan does not believe he could deal with the headaches and fatigue of a caffeine-free life. Although he had the strength to give up tobacco, he feels powerless in this situation.

As described by Bandura in 1977, the social learning theory became known as the social cognitive theory (SCT) in 1986 (Rosenstock, Strecher, and Becker, 1988). This theory has an environmental as well as an interpersonal component.

SCT acknowledges that humans have influence over their environment. The environment influences the individual and the individual influences the environment. This is known as reciprocal determinism. Human behavior is not merely operant conditioning, as with Pavlov's dogs. People's ability to change the environment is very useful in initiating and maintaining a behavior change so they can adapt the environment to support their new behavior. Human beings also learn from the environment and other people. People can see behavior that they admire and use it as a model.

> Juan knows he can find alternatives to coffee during the workday. He has changed his environment by removing his coffee cup from his desk and staying away from the lunch room and coffee machines during breaks. But, ahhh, not the first cup in the morning. After three weeks of only one cup of coffee each morning, Juan has lunch with his friend Colombo and notices that he asks for decaf. Juan decides to model this behavior and asks for decaf the next morning.

In addition to the dynamic influence of the environment, SCT takes into account the individual's confidence in the new behavior's ability to deliver the desired results. The two most important factors in SCT are outcome expectancies and self-efficacy. Bandura believed that a person's behavior is influenced by his or her personal belief that a certain behavior will, in fact, produce a desired effect or outcome. Only when armed with this belief can the individual move on to believing he or she has the competence and ability to perform the specific behavior.

Self-efficacy beliefs vary from situation to situation. For example, smokers who feel confident that they can refrain from smoking in a movie theater may have no confidence that they can do the same at a party or bar. As health behavior change agents, we must help build situational self-efficacy within the individuals we are helping to change. Identifying when they have high self-efficacy and in which situations they have doubts will help them prepare for dangerous situations where a relapse to the old unwanted action may occur. A second strategy is for individuals to alter the dangerous situation to ensure success; for example, they might arrange to toast with sparkling cider rather than champagne at a wedding reception. Prediction of success may be made by asking individuals whether they have a high or low confidence in their ability to perform a specific behavior in a specific situation. Self-efficacy ratings have proven useful in predicting how long individuals can maintain new behavior and in which situations they risk failure.

Just because individuals believe they can make a behavior change is not enough. They must also believe that as a result of making the change there will be a benefit. In Juan's case, he couldn't reduce his caffeine any further until he believed that cutting down his caffeine consumption would benefit his heart health. Health care practitioners can do much to help individuals align these beliefs so that behavior change can be successful.

Pre-adult Health Decision-Making Model

Virginia, fourteen years old, runs with a fast crowd. She has had the sex education class required at her middle school. She doesn't "exactly" intend to have sex with Richard but things get, you know, going, and well. . . .

The pre-adult health decision-making model (PAHDM) looks at how adolescents make health-related decisions (Langer and Warheit, 1992). It is evident to those who have worked with teenagers that they do not make decisions in the same manner as adults. As the public health issues of STDs, HIV, teen pregnancy, drug and alcohol abuse,and smoking reach an ever younger group, it serves us well to look briefly at this model.

It comes as no surprise that teens are greatly influenced by their peers in the area of personal health practices. Adolescents take cues from society at large and then model their beliefs and knowledge in their behavior. One thing is clear: traditional behavior change approaches may not work when dealing with a younger group. The usual risk-reduction programs providing information may not take into account the social and peer orientation of the teen.

Fortunately for Virginia, all the girls in her crowd think it's cool to carry condoms with them. So when things with Richard heat up she is prepared. She knows a girl in gym class that got pregnant last term.

The PAHDM suggests that much like the area of perceived susceptibility from the health belief model, if the teen does not feel personally at risk the information might be seen as irrelevant. Central to any teen program is the concept that adolescence is a phenomenon in progress and will end with time. However, most teen decisions are strongly influenced by their reference group. Concern is that while teens break bonds with their parents, establish a new peer group, and hone their new identity, they may make poor health-related decisions that will affect the rest of their life.

The PAHDM takes components from the health belief model, the social cognitive theory, the theory of reasoned action, and the model of decision making proposed by Janis and Mann (not covered in this chapter).

The PAHDM addresses the following five coping patterns:

- Ignoring the message and continuing the risky behavior

- Adopting the recommended behavior

- Procrastinating or rationalizing to postpone or avoid making a health-related decision

- Panicking and overreacting to the risk at hand

- Gathering all the information and weighing the alternatives before making a choice (Langer and Warheit, 1992)

Virginia finds that she is too shy to ask Richard to use the condom so she convinces herself she won't get pregnant by having sex just once. Luckily, Richard suggests using one himself.

The bottom line is that with adolescents and adults alike the environment or community plays a large role in the health behavior decision-making process (Padula, 1996). Creating social norms of healthy habits is central to creating a healthier population.

Population-Based Models

As we have seen in many of the previous models, an individual's actions are based in part on external cues, on external calls to action, and to some extent on the peer group and community norms and expectations. It is in this context that we take a look at one community- or population-based behavior change model.

The notion of using a media message or a population-based campaign to influence health behavior is very useful, as demonstrated in the cues-to-action component of the health behavior model. Public service campaigns reach a wide base of people and can communicate sufficient health information to create a tide of behavioral awareness. In the early 1980s, McGuire (1981), a communications expert, described twelve steps in the sequence of events spanning exposure to behavior change:

1. Exposure to the information (exposure)
2. Paying attention to the information (attending)
3. Becoming interested in the information (liking)
4. Learning and understanding the information (what)
5. Gaining the skills necessary (how)
6. Changing one's attitude regarding the information (yielding)
7. Storing the content and one's agreement in memory (internalizing)
8. Information and retrieval (seeking-gathering)
9. Decision making (preparation)
10. Adopting new behavior in accord with the decision (action)
11. Reinforcing the desired behavior (maintenance)
12. Postbehavioral consolidation (termination)

Although this model has many salient points, in modern society everyone is bombarded with thousands of messages each day—

some positive and others negative. Getting the attention of a targeted group is a huge challenge for public health professionals. However, in concert with the other behavior change programs, it is necessary to have a social marketing type communication of health policy and goals. Many examples can be seen in the underage tobacco prevention programs on the airwaves today.

Once you get the attention of the individual, there are still many steps to complete before change is adopted. Using public service announcements and community campaigns will augment the impact of the behavior change program.

Another communitywide health program model is PRECEDE-PROCEED developed by Green and Kreuter. Originally this model was designed to help health educators identify all the factors that are needed in planning a population-based program. (See Chapter Four for further discussion of this model.)

Conclusion

It appears that health-related behavior is too complex to be explained or influenced by any one model. Health behavior changes do not occur as a single event but as a lifelong process of personal survival. Compounding this situation is the reality that personal health status is not created in isolation. Public health issues of poverty, politics, access, and priorities in society at large all play a role in the health of citizens. It is in communities where the most effective social change can take place and have a public health impact. Learning from the seminal work of Saul Alinsky (1972) and others in the area of community organization, we can adapt two of these principles:

- Disorganize the status quo. Start where the client is.

- Identify and freeze targets. Issue selection should be local, specific, and winnable.

This chapter has shown that health behavior can be influenced at many intersection points where there is opportunity for an intervention—those needed "teachable moments." Health care providers have the responsibility to arm themselves with as much data and tools as possible and then analyze a unique set of variables—person, place, time, circumstance, and the individual's preferred learning style—before choosing which techniques to use. When it comes to catalyzing a health behavior change, the mantra is try, try, try again until you succeed.

Remember that health professionals are change agents facilitating an individual's self-directed behavior change process. Contributing to building self-efficacy in individuals may well be the most important skill you can teach. An encouraging word or praise from a health care provider goes a very long way (Seligman, 1990). Gaining the belief that one has control over one's own health status is a powerful motivator. Furthermore, in the areas of self-managed care, active participation on the health care team increases the tendency to be active in compliance of medical regimen.

This chapter has provided a look at the fundamental health behavior change models that can provide a foundation on which health educators and health care practitioners may build. When designing health behavior change programs, it may very well be that health professionals will choose elements of wisdom from each of these basic models to construct a usable new framework for the future.

References

Ajzen, I. "From Intention to Actions: A Theory of Planned Behavior." In J. Kuhl and J. Beckmann (eds.), *Action-Control: From Cognition to Behavior.* Heidelberg: Springer, 1985, pp. 11–30.

Alinsky, S. D. *Rules for Radicals.* New York: Random House, 1972.

Blue, C. L. "The Predictive Capacity of the Theory of Reasoned Action and the Theory of Planned Behavior in Exercise Research: An Integrated Literature Review." *Research in Nursing and Health,* 1995, 18, 105–121.

Bond, G. G., Aiken, L. S., and Somerville, S. C. "The Health Belief Model and Adolescents with Insulin Dependent Diabetes Mellitus." *Health Psychology,* 1992, 11(3), 190–198.

Champion, V. L. "The Relationship of Breast Self-Examination to Health Belief Model Variables." *Research in Nursing and Health*, 1997, 10, 375–382.

Courneya, K. S. "Understanding Readiness for Regular Physical Activity in Older Individuals: An Application of the Theory of Planned Behavior." *Health Psychology*, 1995, 14(1), 80–87.

Courneya, K. S., and McAuley, E. "Cognitive Mediators of the Social Influence–Exercise Adherence Relationship: A Test of the Theory of Planned Behavior." *Journal of Behavioral Medicine*, 1995, 18(5).

Disease State Management Sourcebook, 1998. A resource guide to chronic care programs. New York: Faulkner & Gray, 1998.

Dishman, R. K. *Exercise Adherence: Its Impact on Public Health.* Champaign, Ill.: Human Kinetics, 1988.

Ferguson, T. *The No Nag, No Guilt, Do It Your Own Way, Guide to Quitting Smoking.* New York: Ballantine, 1987.

Ferrini, R., Edelstein, S., and Barrett-Connor, E. "The Association Between Health Beliefs and Health Behavior Change in Older Adults." *Preventive Medicine*, 1994, 23, 1–5.

Glanz, K., Lewis, F. M., and Rimer, B. K. (eds.). *Health Behavior and Health Education: Theory, Research, and Practice.* (2nd ed.) San Francisco: Jossey-Bass, 1997.

Glasser, W. M. *Positive Addiction.* New York: HarperCollins, 1976.

Godin, G., and Kok, G. "The Theory of Planned Behavior: A Review of Its Applications to Health-Related Behaviors." *American Journal of Health Promotion*, Nov./Dec. 1996, 11(2).

Grodner, M. "Using the Health Belief Model for Bulimia." *Journal of American College Health*, Nov. 1991, 40(3), 107–112.

Hedeker, D., Flay, B. R., and Petraitis, J. "Estimating Individual Influences of Behavioral Intentions: An Application of Random-Effects Modeling to the Theory of Reasoned Action." *Journal of Consulting and Clinical Psychology*, 1996, 64(1), 109–120.

Jones, S. L., Jones, P. K., and Katz, J. "Compliance in Acute and Chronic Patients Receiving a Health Belief Model Intervention in the Emergency Department." *Social Science Medicine*, 1991, 32(10), 1183–1189.

Kaplan, R. M., Sallis, J. F., and Patterson, T. L. *Health and Human Behavior.* New York: McGraw-Hill, 1993.

Kolb, D. *Experiential Learning.* Englewood Cliffs, N.J.: Prentice Hall, 1984.

Langer, L. M., and Warheit, G. J. "The Pre-adult Health Decision-Making Model: Linking Decision-Making Directness/Orientation to Adolescent Health Related Attitudes and Behaviors." *Adolescence*, winter 1992, 27(108).

Marlatt, A. G., and Gordon, J. R. *Relapse Prevention Maintenance Strategies in the Treatment of Addictive Behaviors*. New York: Guilford Press, 1985.

McGinnis, J. M. "The Role of Patient Education in Achieving National Health Objectives." *Patient Education Quarterly*, 1993, 21, 1–3.

McGuire, W. J. "Theoretical Foundations of Campaigns." In R. E. Rice and W. J. Paisly (eds.), *Public Communication Campaigns*. Beverly Hills, Calif.: Sage, 1981, pp. 41–70.

Mechanic, D. *Handbook of Health, Healthcare, and the Health Professions*. New York: Free Press, 1983.

Mechanic, D. "Sociological Dimensions of Illness Behavior." *Social Science Medicine*, 1995, 41(9), 1207–1216.

Padula, C. "Older Couples' Decision Making on Health Issues." *Western Journal of Nursing Research*, 1996, 18(6), 675–687.

Prochaska, J. O., Norcross, J. C., and DiClemente, C. C. *Changing for Good*. New York: Avon, 1984.

Rosenstock, I. M., Strecher, V. J., and Becker, M. H. "Social Learning Theory and the Health Belief Model." *Health Education Quarterly*, summer 1988, 15(2), 175–183.

Schafer, R. B., Keith, P. M., and Schafer, E. "Predicting Fat in Diets of Marital Partners Using the Health Belief Model." *Journal of Behavioral Medicine*, 1995, 18(5).

Schiaffino, K. M., and Cea, C. D. "Assessing Chronic Illness Representations: The Implicit Models of Illness Questionnaire." *Journal of Behavioral Medicine*, 1995, 18(6).

Scicchitano, J., and others. "Illness Behavior and Somatization in General Practice." *Journal of Psychosomatic Research*, 1996, 41(3), 247–254.

Seligman, M.E.P. *Learned Optimism*. New York: Knopf, 1990.

Strecher, V. J. "Goal Setting As a Strategy for Health Behavior Change." *Health Education Quarterly*, May 1995, 22(2), 190–200.

U.S. Preventive Services Task Force. *Guide to Clinical Preventive Services*. (2nd ed.) Baltimore: Williams & Wilkins, 1996.

Velicer, W. F., Rossi, J. S., Prochaska, J. O., and DiClemente, C. C. "A Criterion Measurement Model for Health Behavior Change." *Addictive Behaviors*, 1996, 21(5), 555–584.

Watson, D. L., and Thorpe, R. G. *Self-Directed Behavior: Self-Modification for Personal Adjustment*. (7th ed.) Pacific Grove, Calif.: Brooks/Cole, 1997.

Part II

. . . .

From Theory to Practice

The Foundation for Changing Health-Related Behavior

In a field as richly complex as patient behavior, a straightforward application of theoretical models is unlikely to account for necessary subtleties. Instead, the goal should be to cultivate a deeper understanding of why patients behave as they do and then apply that understanding in the development of more effective behavior change tools, interventions, and programs. On this foundation planners can plot a strategy and develop program contents that work for real patients in the real world.

Part One introduced the theories and models that Part Two launches into practice. Part Two looks first at the broader concerns of changing patient behavior and environment and, second, at a familiar technology—the telephone—and its startling effectiveness as a tool for health behavior intervention.

In Chapter Four, Kay Bartholomew, Guy Parcel, Gerjo Kok, and Nell Gottlieb offer step-by-step instructions for planning a theory- and evidence-based disease management program. From standards of practice and needs assessments to program implementation and outcomes measurement, the authors provide an impressive array of practical insights and tools for planning and implementing a coherent program.

Once the program approach and content are determined, one must define the methods for delivering the intervention. In Chapter Five Terry Mason champions the good old telephone as one of the health and disease manager's most powerful tools. Telephone-based interventions have recently seen exponential growth as a medium for behavior change in demand management and disease management systems. Mason reviews the use of telephone-based interventions, including systems featuring voice mailboxes, menu-based prerecorded messages, interactive voice response, and nurse triage lines.

4

. . . .

Changing Behavior and Environment

How to Plan Theory- and Evidence-Based Disease Management Programs

L. Kay Bartholomew, Guy S. Parcel,
Gerjo Kok, Nell H. Gottlieb

T his chapter presents disease management and patient education planning as a specific type of health education and health promotion planning. Techniques from health education and health promotion planners provide a rich resource for those addressing disease management issues. Fundamentally, successful disease management is about change: typically, change in the behavior of the person who has a health problem and, often, change in the social and physical environments as well. A well-planned disease management program will also include strategies for facilitating and reinforcing behavior change in people in the patient's environment such as caretakers and health care providers.

Standards of Practice

Whether health education is taking place in health care settings, schools, the workplace, or community sites, effective population-based programs share certain characteristics. Research has shown that to have the greatest chance of success (an effect on behavior, environment, quality of life, or health status), programs should

- Be epidemiologically based, grounded on data concerning the health problem and its consequences (Green and Kreuter, 1999)

- Take an ecological approach to understanding both the problem and the solution (McLeroy, Bibeau, Steckler, and Glanz, 1988; Stokols, 1996; Richard and others, 1996; Simons-Morton, Simons-Morton, Parcel, and Bunker, 1988)

- Use a program development logic that analyzes the association between behavioral and environmental causes and the health problem itself (Green and Kreuter, 1999)

- Use both social science theory and evidence to build hypotheses about determinants of these behavioral and environmental factors (McLeroy and others, 1995; Cullen, Bartholomew, Parcel, and Kok, 1998; Bartholomew, Parcel and Kok, 1998; Bartholomew, Parcel, Kok, and Gottlieb, 2000)

- Involve the program participants (patients, caretakers, family members) and program users (health care providers) in the planning (Robertson and Minkler, 1994; Minkler, 1997)

- Take into consideration the interaction between cognition, behavior, and environment and between levels of environment (Bandura, 1986; Stokols, 1996; Richard and others, 1996; Minkler, 1997)

- Be tailored both to important determinants of behavior (which may vary among individuals) and to demographic characteristics, such as age or ethnicity (Strecher and others, 1994; Skinner, Strecher, and Hospers, 1994)

Deficits in Patient Education
and Disease Management

These standards of practice may be most often met in health education or health promotion programs in schools, worksites, or the community—sites other than health care. The lack of incorporation of these standards of practice into many disease management programs may be due, oddly enough, to the greater knowledge to be found in the health care setting. The health care milieu is the only one in which there is a preexisting base of extensive expert knowledge of health and illness. At the same time, there is often no comparable expertise in behavioral science. As health care professionals, we may not always recognize that learning styles differ among people or that patient education requires a different approach than student education. Faced with the needs of patients, a common question in the halls of health care is "What does the patient need to know?" or "What do I need to tell them?" This is the information transfer approach—seeing education as communication of information from health care provider to patient. As pointed out in previous chapters, we cannot expect to have effective program outcomes without also using effective behavior change methods.

Planning for Effective Programs

Incorporating behavioral science into the planning of disease management programs can seem a complex task, even a daunting one. One must consider several theories of varying familiarity, use empirical findings from a wide-ranging literature, and identify what new information is needed from program participants and implementers. How do we find a way through the maze? Know when to use theory in making decisions and what theory or theories to use? Decide which intervention methods will be effective in influencing behavior? How can we move from program goals and objectives to specific intervention strategies? Link program design with planning for program implementation? Because behavior occurs in an ecological context, we must also address changing the environment—but how?

Over the past twenty years, significant enhancements have been made to the conceptual base and practice of health promotion, especially in needs assessment and program evaluation. However, the field has been slow to specify the processes involved in program design and development. Advances have been made in the application of behavioral and social science theories to intervention design (Glanz, Lewis, and Rimer, 1997; Maibach and Parrot, 1995), but even in this regard the processes for theory application have not typically been made explicit in the research or practice literature.

We present in this chapter a brief description of a framework, Intervention Mapping, which the authors of this chapter have created to guide program planners through the steps needed to move from an ecological analysis of the problem to an integrated, effective disease management or patient education program (Bartholomew, Parcel, Kok, and Gottlieb, 2000; Bartholomew, Parcel, and Kok, 1998). Intervention Mapping has been used to develop and evaluate a number of health promotion and disease management programs (Bartholomew and others, 1991; Cullen, Bartholomew, Parcel, and Kok, 1998; Murray, Kelder, Parcel, and Orpinas, 1998; Bartholomew and others, 2000).

Analysis of Needs and Capacities

The needs assessment literature, particularly Green and Kreuter's (1999) PRECEDE model, has helped the health education and health promotion community focus on behavior change rather than on simple information transfer. The PRECEDE model provides a framework for linking health and quality-of-life outcomes with their behavioral and environmental causes. It has also provided some useful guidance about how to think about the determinants of these behavioral and environmental causes.

A complete needs assessment has two components:

- A scientific epidemiological assessment that includes both behavioral and social analyses of the patients or at-risk group and their health problems (The epidemiological and behavioral diagnoses are what most people mean when they use the term *needs assessment*.)

- A capacity component that investigates the resources and strengths of the patients in the group and their caregivers and health care providers

Epidemiological, Behavioral, Environmental, and Educational Diagnoses

The first part of a needs assessment is a systematic study of quality of life and health status and of the factors that influence them, such as health behavior and environment. Such an assessment may include consideration of physiological risk factors and behavioral and environmental risks to health, even if the actual health problem has not yet manifested itself; for example, with respect to cardiovascular disease, we might wish to evaluate the prevalence of high cholesterol levels (a physiological risk factor), eating high-fat foods (a behavioral risk factor), and poor access to a healthy diet (an environmental risk factor). Finally, we must consider the factors related to these behavioral and environmental contributors to health problems and health risks.

Capacity Component

The study of a patient or at-risk group from a capacity perspective (their resources and strengths) rounds out the needs assessment. Addressing the capacity component gives two advantages to the resulting program plan. First, being mindful of a patient group's strengths helps us judge capability to form instrumental partnerships

with health care providers and other professionals; such partnerships are essential to avoid the trap of one-way communication.
Second, a focus on patient competencies and resources from the
outset of program planning keeps us mindful during program development and implementation of the need to enhance those capaci-
ties. A goal of every disease management or patient education
program should be to leave the members of the intervention group
not simply doing what they have been told to do but more skillful
in meeting their own needs for disease-related learning (whether
information or skill training) and more skillful in planning their
own interventions.

Using the PRECEDE Framework

One of the strengths of the PRECEDE model is that it reminds the
planner of both important predictors and important consequences
of the health problem. It also offers an incisive way to organize the
information obtained in the needs assessment. The first task in the
needs assessment is designating the at-risk population. It must be a
group with a definable boundary and shared characteristics. Typically a group has a risk factor or health problem in common; for
example, high blood pressure, obesity, cystic fibrosis, cardiovascular
disease, or AIDS. Sometimes we are interested in a subgroup of a
larger population, such as people with asthma who frequently present to the emergency department (ED). The population may be
defined by a number of variables; for example, children with asthma
who live in the inner city and are at risk for high ED use. The more
well-defined the intervention population, the more adequate the
needs assessment will be (Soriano, 1995; Witkin and Altschuld,
1995; Gilmore, Campbell, and Becker, 1989).

The PRECEDE model is famous for one peculiarity: it is created
backwards. Information is filled in from right to left instead of from
left to right, as is typical in the English language. Using Exhibit 4.1
as an example, we begin with the outcome at the far right: the
epidemiological assessment of quality-of-life indicators such as

Exhibit 4.1.   PRECEDE Model for Pediatric Asthma.

Educational Diagnosis →	*Behavioral and Environmental Analyses* →	*Epidemiological and Social Analyses*
Predisposing Factors	*Behavioral Factors*	*Health Outcomes and Quality of Life*
Behavioral capability	Symptom monitoring	
Self-efficacy	• Directly (symptoms)	Health status
Outcome expectations	• Objectively (peak flow)	Symptoms
Attribution	Environmental monitoring	Hospitalizations
Value placed	Medication use	Emergency visits
on independent	• Control meds	Child's adaptive
management	• Relief meds	functioning
	• Premedicating	School performance
Enabling Factors	Provider access	School absenteeism
	• Acute situations	Functional status
Access to medical care	• Regular appointments	
Access to training	Environmental tobacco	
Parent/child	smoke, other allergen	
self-regulation skills	exposure	
Parent/child		
asthma-specific skills		
Skills needed to		
transfer tasks to		
children as appropriate	*Environmental Factors*	
	Indoor irritants and	
Reinforcing Factors	allergens—home and school	
	• Sprays, powders, perfumes,	
Social reinforcement	insecticides	
from provider and	• Dust mites, cockroaches,	
school	pet dander, mold	
	Outdoor irritants and	
	allergens	
	• Air pollutants (particulate	
	and ozone)	
	• Allergens (pollen)	
	Medical care	
	• Objective measurement of	
	lung function	
	• Prescription of control	
	medications	
	• Formulation and	
	discussion of action plan	

absenteeism, performance, and self-esteem. From there we step back (move left) to indicators and dimensions of the health problem itself, which are the cause of the quality-of-life issues. Health indicators include disability, morbidity, mortality, and physiological risk factors. Their dimensions may be expressed in terms of distribution, duration, incidence, intensity, or prevalence. (For a more complete list of possible indicators, see Green and Kreuter, 1999.)

Exhibit 4.1 shows a compressed PRECEDE framework for children with asthma. The arrows indicate causality, *not* the order in which the information was determined. At the far right, health status indicators for asthma include symptoms, hospitalizations, and emergency visits; quality-of-life indicators include the burden of the disease on the individual as well as on organizations and society at large. Society's interest starts here, for example with the cost of inappropriate use of the ED.

However, the analysis should not be limited to any one viewpoint. Understanding the outcomes from a number of perspectives can help a planner conceptualize motivational aspects of the disease outcomes. For instance, the health care provider may be interested in decreased ED usage; the child's family may be more interested in increasing the child's school attendance (and so decreasing a parent's absenteeism or tardiness at work). This multiple-perspective analysis may also point to such collaborators in the disease management process as school nurses and administrators, who may be willing to implement a program that is specifically planned to have a positive impact on school attendance. A good question to ask here is, who cares about these outcomes? Those who care—for whatever personal or impersonal reason—are stakeholders in the problem and therefore possible partners in the intervention. Such partnership may take the form of funding, providing a site, or lending moral support to the intervention program.

Having addressed quality of life and health outcomes, the planner moves to the left in the PRECEDE framework (to the middle column) and makes two more lists: behavioral and environmental factors. "Environment" means both the social and the physical factors that can contribute to health problems directly or through behavior. In addition, all the "ecological levels" of environment must be considered: the interpersonal and organizational levels, the community, and society at large (Richard and others, 1996).

Note that behavioral and environmental factors often interact and reinforce one another. In conducting a behavioral analysis, the planner asks what individuals could do that would either decrease their risk of having the health problem or, in the case of secondary or tertiary prevention, decrease their risk of disability or death as a result of the health problem. In the environmental analysis, we ask what conditions of the environment are related to the health problem directly or to its behavioral causes. Asthma is a particularly compelling example of an environmental analysis because elements of both the physical environment (indoor and outdoor allergens and irritants) and the health care environment (the behavior of health care providers) impact health directly and have an effect on the behavior required of children and their families in managing the disease.

In this particular example, the behavioral risk factors include being around environmental tobacco smoke and other triggers and failing to monitor symptoms, use medication, and seek consultation with health care providers. The environmental factors are in two subsets: the child's physical environment (indoor and outdoor irritants and allergens) and his or her health care environment (for example, the lack of an asthma action plan).

We must not dismiss any factors as a matter of course. That which seems blindingly obvious is sometimes the most often ignored. For example, the physician guidelines from the expert panel of the National Asthma Education and Prevention Program focus on three main areas: diagnosis with objective measurement of lung function and categorization of severity; control of the inflammatory process with medication for persistent asthma; and patient-physician communication, including formulation and discussion of an asthma action plan (*Expert Panel Report 2*, 1997). All three of these areas are problematic in most communities. Preliminary estimates in one large urban area are that 62 percent of elementary-school children with asthma are unknown to school nurses (Tortolero and others, in preparation). Underprescription of anti-inflammatory medication may be as high as 89 percent for inner-city children (Finkelstein and others, 1995; Lieu and others, 1997; Homer and others, 1996). In one large city among children with persistent moderate-to-severe asthma who were referred for specialty care, fewer than 16 percent had been prescribed anti-inflammatory medications (Sockrider and others, 1998). The lack of behavior-focused patient education, such as use of action plans, is documented in the work of Dawson and others (1995). Under these medical care conditions, a planner might choose as appropriate intervention groups the medical care providers for these children as well as the at-risk children themselves. The behavior of the physician can be a "high-impact leverage point"—a place to intervene that will garner the most change for the least effort and also produce change across ecological levels (Stokols, 1996). For example, getting physicians to use action plans might influence both physician prescribing behavior and patient adherence to medication regimens.

Having completed behavioral and environmental analyses, the planner moves to the left to the first column in the PRECEDE framework and makes a list of the factors that may influence behavior and environment (which in turn create the health problems and quality-of-life outcomes). We do this by asking in three different ways why a family would perform the designated behavior. First, what are the predisposing factors (the personal motivational factors)? Second, what are the enabling factors (the facilitators outside the individual)? Third, what are the reinforcing factors (events that happen after the behavior is initiated that make the behavior more frequent)? These hypothetical determinants—"hypothetical" because the evidence is usually statistical association rather than causation—are the link to the intervention.

At this point, the planner is building a risk model: What are the (hypothetical) determinants of the behavioral and environmental risks? However, in the development of interventions, the planner will switch the model from risk to health promotion in order to address health promoting behavior and environments. The planner will again ask a question about determinants: What are the hypothetical determinants of the health promoting behavior and environmental conditions? To answer this question and many others in theory-based intervention planning we suggest several core processes that we present here before moving into the steps of Intervention Mapping.

Obtaining Needed Data and Information

A complete needs assessment requires a great deal of information. Where does it come from? Once we have a preliminary definition of the at-risk population, we begin with a literature search. What do others know about the health problem and its causes and management? We may need to go beyond our usual sources of information, for example, perform a literature search using CINAHL (the Cumulative Index to Nursing and Allied Health Literature) as well as MEDLINE or CHID (the federal government's Combined Health Information Database). If little appears on the specific health problem, research similar health problems. We may need to think laterally about what might be similar. What kinds of health problems have similar intervention groups? Have similar impacts on quality of life (such as impaired mobility)? Require similar skills in self-management (for example, monitoring symptoms or other data)?

We must also find appropriate administrative data, such as the size of the at-risk group and the health care utilization patterns of this population. Then, and equally important, we must ask questions of members of the intervention group and of the people in their environment. What is involved in managing this disease? What problems does it cause in their lives? What barriers do they encounter in attempting to live as healthfully as possible? This is subjective information, but it is no less important than objective data. One needs both an objective assessment of the difference between current and optimal status and a subjective assessment of what the problems and needs mean to the persons with the health problem. To comprehend both the objective and the subjective perspectives, the planner must use both qualitative and quantitative data. Quantitative methods, such as surveys, utilization statistics, and disease registries, allow us to estimate the incidence and prevalence of the health problem and its related behaviors. However, to understand the problems and their determinants from the perspective of the people involved, there are no substitutes for such qualitative methods as interviews (Bauman and Adair, 1992) and focus groups (Basch, 1987; Kreuger, 1988).

Core Processes for Intervention Mapping

How do we use theory and empirical evidence to establish hypothetical determinants? How do we use theory and evidence to answer other intervention-related questions, such as which methods to use to create change in determinants? Veen (1985) offers useful approaches for using theory and empirical evidence. As suggested by Veen, we ask first, Why do (or would) people do the behavior of interest? For example, why would parents of a child with asthma give their child control (anti-inflammatory) medications? We then brainstorm possible explanations. Making a list of provisional answers to such a question is a creative process that involves free association, lateral thinking, and a fair amount of empathy.

In formulating these provisional explanations, planners unavoidably will bring specific theoretical knowledge to the table, whether consciously or not. The theories can be illuminating and helpful, but the list of possible determinants should not be limited to either explicitly data-based or theory-based items. In brainstorming possible determinants, the task is not to generate or test a particular theory (the problem-of-the-theory approach), but rather to see how many theories might help in developing comprehensive and productive answers to the question (the theory-of-the-problem approach). In this respect, all theories are right.

Having created a list, we check the provisional explanations against further possible answers that may lie in the empirical literature. A topic search will garner both theoretical and empirical explanation. To continue the pediatric asthma example, the planning group attempted to answer the question "Why would parents give their children control medication?" by looking for what others had found regarding medication-taking in asthma. They found evidence of the underprescribing of anti-inflammatory medication and added this to the list they had compiled during the brainstorming session. In this topical approach to the literature, broadening the topic to include related issues and target populations is important. Mindful of this, the group also looked for information on medication used for other chronic diseases, such as diabetes (Glasgow, McCaul, and Schafer, 1986). In this way they found the concept of the patient's ideas about disease causation as a predictor of adherence, and they added this concept to their list. In reviewing the literature, the planner will find new explanations, cross some items off the preliminary list, and find new questions that require additional research (Kok and others, 1996).

The next approach to the literature is to look for theories that will add to the list of provisional explanations. There are three helpful approaches to searching the literature for applicable theories—issues, concept, and general theories.

Beginning with the *issue* approach, the planner can look again at the literature in reference to the subject or issue, but this time with an eye to finding theoretical constructs to the specific health or behavior problem. For instance, planners working on the problem of parents not giving asthma medications found a considerable number of studies that used variables from social cognitive theory (Bandura, 1986) as predictors of medication-taking behavior: skills, self-efficacy (confidence in being able to give the medication correctly), and outcome expectations (belief that giving the medication will result in better health for the child and will not cause bad side effects).

The *concept* approach enables the planner to track backward from concepts on the provisional list to theoretical constructs and then on to the parent theories. Exploring a theoretical construct may help to explicate the meaning of a concept on the provisional list. For instance, the pediatric asthma group began with "perception of symptoms" on their provisional list. By this they did not mean noticing the symptoms, but the attitude and beliefs of parents about the importance and meaning of symptoms. They found a similar concept in the constructs of severity and susceptibility in the health belief model (Becker, 1974; Janz and Becker, 1984). On further discussion, the group was able to articulate that what they meant by "perception of symptoms" was first, the parents' recognizing that persistent symptoms indicate a serious problem and second, their acknowledging their child's susceptibility to asthma episodes. They changed "perception of symptoms" to read "perception that low-level persistent symptoms are serious" and "perception that if the inflammation underlying low-level symptoms is not controlled, the child is susceptible to an asthma episode." Notice how much more precise and detailed the revised determinants are. The greater the precision and detail, the more likely it is that appropriate ways can be found to affect the determinant.

Many times the parent theory behind a construct will prove to have other germane constructs in addition to those that brought us to the theory in the first place. For instance, when the construct "perception of symptoms" led the asthma group to the health belief model, the planners found another useful construct: barriers. They determined they already had two barriers on their list: physicians' not prescribing anti-inflammatory medication and the family's inability to pay for the doctor visit or medications. What other barriers belonged on the list? The question led them to adding "inaccurate advice of family and friends" and "lack of child's cooperation" as possible additional barriers.

With the third approach, *general theories*, the planner can look at the question through the lens of a determinants theory or a change theory, as appropriate. For instance, if the question concerns determinants of behavior, we might go to social cognitive theory or the health belief model if we have not already considered them. This is the time for members of the planning group to review their favorite theories and see if they have anything useful to add to the list.

The penultimate step in checking our preliminary hypotheses is to obtain qualitative information as to their relative importance to the intervention group, using focus groups and interviews. In other words, we go to the source and ask. Some items, perhaps all, will be confirmed as important, and we will find out how each construct is expressed in the intervention group (both the details of how it presents and the language they use to describe it). Some items may turn out to be irrelevant to our particular intervention group. We may also discover additional determinants that need to be added to the list.

The last step is to organize the results. We can rate the hypothetical determinants on two dimensions: the importance of the determinant as indicated by association between the proposed determinant and the behavior and the changeability of the determinant within the scope of the project. Those that are both important and changeable should be the ones addressed. We would also categorize the determinants as personal (internal to the members of the intervention group) or external (from some level of the environment, from interpersonal to societal). This last issue is important in maintaining clarity in intervention design, as an intervention directed solely to the at-risk group will be unlikely to have much effect on environmental factors.

Intervention Mapping

Intervention Mapping is a step-by-step, task-by-task process for moving from the problem assessment through program design, production, implementation, and evaluation. It is an approach that coaches the planner through the process of combining theory and evidence to produce an intervention that is effective in changing behavior and environmental conditions. Intervention Mapping is composed of five steps, each of which includes multiple tasks. At the end of each step, the planner has a concrete product that then serves as the foundation for the next step. Approached on a task-by-task, step-by-step basis, Intervention Mapping can make an otherwise daunting and confusing task approachable and performable.

The five steps of Intervention Mapping are

1. Creating matrices of proximal program objectives
2. Arriving at an appropriate list of theory-based methods and practical strategies
3. Writing a program plan
4. Developing a plan for adoption and implementation of the program
5. Writing an evaluation plan for the program

The Matrices

The first step of Intervention Mapping is creating matrices of proximal program objectives—what it is we want the program to accomplish in the short term. To develop these matrices, we have to know the following:

1. The behavior and environmental conditions that need to be changed
2. The specific components of the behavior or environmental change; that is, what someone has to do to perform the health behavior or to make the environmental change
3. What personal factors (within individuals) and what external factors (outside of individuals) are related to the performance of these actions (hypothetical determinants)

Specifying Behavioral and Environmental Changes

The first task of Intervention Mapping, therefore, is stating in explicit terms the changes in behavior and environment that are the purpose of the program. Referring to Exhibit 4.1 on page 79, we might list explicit changes in the behavior of parents, children, and health care providers (the health care environment). An even more comprehensive program would target the physical environment of the home and school as well (Tyrrell and others, in preparation). Planners must be careful not to allow themselves to be too easily discouraged about what is practical; as noted above, a careful delineation of those who are stakeholders in the problem may yield unexpected leverage points for change.

Defining Performance Objectives

Once a planner knows what the intervention is intended to change, the next task is to write detailed performance objectives. A performance objective is what an individual needs to do in order to perform a specific health behavior. A performance objective for an environmental condition specifies what someone needs to do to change the condition and how he or she will do it. From an ecological perspective, individual behavior has multiple levels of context within the environment, from interpersonal through organizational and community systems. When addressing environmental change, planners should look at the various ecological levels and designate the people or roles who are responsible for the environmental condition or who are in a position to change it. If the issue is availability of adequate asthma action plans, for instance, one must consider the health care provider and other staff.

Exhibit 4.2 shows a partial set of the performance objectives for the health care providers of children with asthma, and Exhibit 4.3 presents the performance objectives for children and their caretakers with respect to monitoring symptoms and taking

Exhibit 4.2.   Sample Pediatric Asthma Performance Objectives for Health Care Providers.

Diagnosis

The health care provider will

1. Establish diagnosis using NAEPP assessment and modified severity guidelines
   - Establish findings from medical history that increase probability of asthma
   - Establish findings from physical examination of upper respiratory tract, chest, and skin that increase probability of asthma
   - Determine episodic symptoms of airflow obstruction and reversibility
   - Exclude alternative diagnoses
2. Establish severity by NAEPP guidelines: mild intermittent, mild persistent, moderate persistent, or severe persistent
   - Establish symptom prevalence and duration; establish frequency of nighttime symptoms
   - Establish lung function (predicted value for FEV_1 or personal best PEF)

Action Plan

The health care provider will

1. Agree on treatment goals with child and family
   - Ask what child would like to do but can't because of asthma and make it a goal
   - Explain that child should sleep through the night and require no or minimal emergency department visits or missed school
   - Explain that child should feel well and maintain normal activities and normal or near-normal lung function
2. Provide action plan
   - Fill in control medication (after fitting daily medication regimen into child's routine)
   - Explain to child and parents how to discover and avoid triggers
   - Explain to child how to watch for early warning signs and asthma symptoms
   - Fill in rescue plan
   - Follow up with child and parents on performance of action plan at each visit

Exhibit 4.3.   Sample Pediatric Asthma Performance Objectives for Families.

Monitoring

The child (or parent of a young child) will directly monitor symptoms of asthma

- Watch for current symptoms and compare to healthy state
- Watch for prevalence and monitor for changing prevalence
- Report symptoms to parents
- Note symptoms on action plan

Control Medications

The child (or parent of a young child) will take control medications according to action plan

- Plan schedule for control medication
- Continue control medications when symptoms are not present
- Report to physician the effects of control medications

control medication. The needs assessment yielded a general behavior: monitoring for symptoms of asthma. The performance objective breaks this behavior down into its component parts: watching for current symptoms and comparing to a healthy state; watching for and monitoring changes in prevalence of symptoms; for children, reporting symptoms to parents; noting symptoms on the action plan. This is what is meant by directly monitoring for symptoms of asthma. This is one of the tasks in which theory can be of value because a given behavior may have many ways of being broken down into its constituent parts. In the case of asthma, we used Clark and Zimmerman's (1990) analysis of the metacognitive processes necessary for self-regulation: monitoring the situation, comparing to a standard, identifying a problem, planning solutions, trying them out, and evaluating the results. Another contribution from the theoretical literature is the use of coping theory (Lazarus and Folkman, 1984) to augment an understanding of disease management behavior. For example, Exhibit 4.4 illustrates how, in a cystic fibrosis family education program, coping theory

Exhibit 4.4.   Performance Objectives for Coping with Cystic Fibrosis Disease Management

Members of a family of a child with cystic fibrosis (CF) will use coping strategies to manage problems related to CF. They will

1. Recognize need to cope with CF
   - Accept CF as the medical diagnosis (e.g., genetics, prognosis, variable course)
   - Acknowledge potential extent of the physical effects of CF
   - Acknowledge that disease-related problems may occur at any time
   - Recognize need for adjustment by child and family to the demands of self-care
   - Accept the occurrence of emotional distress to the child and family as a periodic consequence of CF
2. Appraise situations for potential problems related to CF
   - Identify sources of stress
   - Identify signs of personal and family stress
   - Estimate likelihood of undesirable outcomes from stressful situations
3. Generate multiple coping alternatives, including categories of action, stopping action, information seeking, and thinking or feeling about things differently
   - Acknowledge the value of using a variety of coping strategies (flexibility)
   - Generate alternatives to solve problems, including strategies of seeking information and social support
   - Generate alternatives to ameliorate emotional distress, such as seeking distraction and social support or practicing anxiety management
4. Use selected alternatives from coping strategies generated
   - Use a variety of strategies to solve problems
   - Use a variety of strategies to ameliorate emotional distress
5. Evaluate effectiveness of coping strategies used
   - Judge whether problem has been solved
   - Judge whether new problems have been created through application of coping strategies
   - Judge whether emotional distress has been reduced
   - Recycle to appraisal if coping strategy is not judged effective

was used to specify exactly how a family might effectively cope with contingencies of disease management (Bartholomew and others, 1993).

Creating the Matrices

After performance objectives are written and important and changeable determinants are proposed, the planner can create the matrices of proximal program objectives, the end product of Step One of Intervention Mapping. As shown in Table 4.1, a matrix is created by entering performance objectives on the left side of the table and determinants across the top. The proximal program objectives are entered into the cells formed at the intersection of each performance objective with each determinant. However, each of the determinants is not likely to be an important influence for every performance objective. One should only write proximal program objectives (either learning or change objectives) for those cells in which the determinant is likely to influence the accomplishment of the performance objective. These cells of proximal program objectives represent the pathways through which the program will have an impact on the health behavior and environmental conditions.

Table 4.1 illustrates *learning objectives*, written by answering the question, "What do the participants in the program need to learn (related to this determinant) to do the performance objective?" and *change objectives*, written by answering the question, "What needs to be changed in the environment (external to the individual) in order for the individual to do the performance objective?"

In an actual program development effort, we would have many pages of matrix as well as additional matrices for parents and different matrices for children at different developmental levels—a matrix for each carefully defined subgroup among the intervention populations. For example, Table 4.2 is a partial matrix for health care providers of children with asthma.

Table 4.1. Pediatric Asthma Matrix for Children and Families.

| | Personal Determinants | | | | External Determinants | |
| | | Perceived | | | | |
Performance Objectives	Outcome Expectations	Seriousness or Susceptibility	Attitudes About Medications	Skills and Self-Efficacy	Barriers— Physician Practices	Barriers—Other
Parent or child takes or gives control medications according to action plan.	Parent or child believes control medications (anti-inflammatories) are important to control underlying inflammation making child susceptible to episodes.	Parent or child • Relates that asthma is chronic disease causing many problems in child's normal activities. • Relates that asthma can still cause deaths.	Parent or child • describes medications for asthma as different from steroids.	Parent or child • Demonstrates ability to use prescribed inhalation device. • Expresses confidence in using prescribed inhalation device.	Anti-inflammatory medication is prescribed for persistent asthma. • Clear messages are given about inflammation and importance of control.	• Children are taught skills for participation.
Parent or child continues control medications when symptoms are not present.	Parent or child expects that control medication is important for child's health even when symptoms have resolved.	Parent or child • Describes level of severity and what this means. • Believes child really has asthma and describes what that is. • Perceives that low-level symptoms are serious.	Parent or child • Describes these medications as having few side effects. • Discusses importance of talking to provider to report symptoms and minimize side effects.	Parent or child • Expresses confidence in ability to report symptoms and side effects to provider. • Increases skill in communicating with provider.		

Table 4.2. Pediatric Asthma Matrix for Health Care Providers—Diagnosis.

	Personal Determinants			External Determinants		
Performance Objectives	Behavioral Capability	Skills and Self-Efficacy	Perceived Social Norms	Outcome Expectations	Office Scheduling Practices
Establish diagnosis using NAEPP Guidelines			Perception that valued colleagues use NAEPP guidelines for assessment of asthma	Belief that diagnosing asthma (vs. treating symptoms) leads to better treatment and resulting outcome	
Establish findings from medical history that increase probability of asthma	Description of how to take history List of findings from history that indicate asthma	Increased confidence and demonstration of ability to extract findings from medical history that increase asthma probability	Perception that valued colleagues establish findings from medical history that increase asthma probability	Belief that specific methods of history taking are important for diagnosis	Office scheduling practices modified for suspected asthma to allow time for thorough diagnostic history
Establish findings from physical examination of upper respiratory tract, chest, and skin that increase probability of asthma	Description of how to establish thorax hyperexpansion, wheezing, prolonged phase of forced exhalation, nasal secretions, mucosal swelling, and so on	Increased confidence and demonstration of ability to extract findings from physical exam that increase asthma probability	Perception that valued colleagues in similar practices establish findings from physical exam that increase asthma probability	Belief that specific methods of physical exam are important for diagnosis	Office scheduling practices modified for suspected asthma to allow time for thorough diagnostic physical

Methods and Strategies

With the matrices of proximal program objectives completed, the planner can move to the second step of Intervention Mapping, matching these proximal program objectives with appropriate theory-based intervention methods and practical strategies. An intervention *method* is a defined process by which, theory postulates, change may occur in the behavior of an individual, small group, or other social structure. Examples of such theory-based methods are modeling, self-monitoring, cognitive-behavioral rehearsal, social comparison, and reattribution, all of which are frequently used to facilitate behavior change.

Whereas a method is a theory-based technique to influence behavior or environmental conditions, a *strategy* is a way of operationalizing an intervention method. Examples of strategies include: for community development, meeting with community members on how to form task forces; for self-monitoring, keeping a diary; for modeling, seeking role-model stories; for commitment, making a pledge; for cognitive-behavioral rehearsal, engaging in self-talk. We must then address the issue of a *delivery* mechanism; for example, to transmit role-model stories, we might use a newsletter, one-on-one coaching sessions, or videotaped vignettes shown in a group session.

Although methods and strategies may be brainstormed at the same moment in the planning process, it is imperative that they are kept conceptually differentiated. Too often, we hear a stream of strategies proposed: "Let's do support groups!" "How about a buddy system?" "We can put it in a training manual." These may be appropriate strategies, but a planner must address the "guts" of the strategy—the change method.

Focusing on Theoretical Methods

To generate a list of methods, the planner can brainstorm responses to the question, "How can the learning and change objectives be influenced?" Again, the processes adapted from Veen (1985) for searching the literature can be great value. Some possible answers to the question "How can these objectives be influenced?" (focusing on the diagnostic behavior of the health care providers of children with asthma) are shown in Table 4.3. It is also appropriate to review the theoretical methods one may have used in the past to see if they might be useful with respect to these determinants as well.

An important part of this step is distinguishing between what is the change-creating part of the intervention and what is the delivery mechanism. In patient education and disease management programs we too often focus on the delivery vehicle—the pamphlet or videotape. In order to create change we must shift the focus to the affective components and address theoretical methods. Unfortunately, this process is not well described in the literature. Disease management professionals may themselves need to adopt the methods of goal setting, commitment, and skill building to begin considering theoretical methods as an integral part of their program planning.

Table 4.3.   **Brainstorming for Methods and Strategies from the Pediatric Asthma Matrix for Health Care Providers—Diagnosis.**

Methods from Theory	Practical Strategies
Modeling	Demonstration by valued colleagues (delivered via videotape)
Skill training	Demonstration, practice, and feedback
Cue to action	• Asthma action plan with child's name • Action plan in hands of family • School nurse reminder
Persuasion	Persuasive expert argument (delivered via videotape)
Social comparison and normative belief change	Presentation of "Who Uses Action Plans" videotape

Methods themselves take a wide variety of forms. Methods to change knowledge, for instance, include chunking, advance organizers, tailoring, and active learning. To change awareness and risk perception, one might choose among reevaluation, fear arousal, and presenting information about personal risk. Methods to change attitudes include self-reevaluation, environmental reevaluation, modeling, and persuasive communication, among many others. Methods to change external determinants include advocacy, community organization, and organizational development. More complete lists of methods and discussions of their uses and possible strategies are available in textbook format (Bartholomew and others, 2000).

Having generated a list of methods, the planner must identify the conditions under which each method is most likely to be effective. For instance, modeling requires active attention from the learner and the learner needs to be reinforced. Fear arousal usually will not result in the desired behavior unless the learner has both high self-efficacy and high outcome expectations; lacking these, it can be counterproductive (Ruiter, Kok, and Abraham, 1999).

Using the winnowed list of methods, the planner will match the proximal program objectives to the methods that seem most suitable for each objective. Note that one method may be appropriate for several objectives and that one objective may be approached by several methods. Creating a table is recommended for organizing the results.

Translating Methods into Strategies

The next task is to translate these methods into practical strategies. Again, we will want to make use of the information already available in the literature as well as brainstorming new possibilities. Here is another instance when the flood of creativity among program planners can be channeled to good effect. Many people have program ideas in mind from the beginning of planning and development, and the task of reining them in until the appropriate moment can be difficult for everyone. We suggest keeping a strategies "parking lot" available on a large newsprint pad throughout the planning process. What strategies had people thought of when they first envisioned what the program might look like? Given the methods and the proximal program objectives, what ideas now come to mind? This is a time to let the brainstorming process run full throttle. One of the fundamental ways that the disease management field progresses is by taking advantage of new strategies and delivery mechanisms. Ten years ago, we could not have even considered a programmable CD-ROM, an electronic mailing list, or a web page. While we do not want to become so enamored of the "toys" that we are sidetracked from solid theory- and evidence-based program planning, neither should we automatically dismiss an idea simply because the technology involved is cutting edge.

Program Materials

Step Three of Intervention Mapping is where, all too often, health professionals *begin* program planning. For many people, it is the most interesting, exciting, and creative part of the entire process. Many people already "know" what the program "should" be at the first planning meeting: "We should send three asthma management videotapes home with the parents—one on control medications, one on relief medications, and one on triggers." "The parents should come to a series of asthma classes. The first is an introduction to asthma, the second is on medications, and the third is on triggers." "We should do a booklet, containing. . . ." Having these thoughts is a sign of creativity; acting on them before the other steps are completed is a sign of derailed planning. The planning group may, indeed, wind up with something that looks very much like one of these ideas. However, without the detailed planning process, they would have no way of knowing the logic model underlying the program. Do the strategies contain the appropriate methods directed toward changing the most likely and important determinants of the most critical behavior and environmental conditions? Is the program directed toward the most important behavioral or environmental targets for change or addressed to the right audiences? Planning may seem tedious to some, but it is extremely cost effective. Nothing is more expensive than a disease management program that does not improve disease management and health status not only because it accrues no benefits to funder or patient but also because it proves to doubters that disease management does not work!

Reviewing Existing Materials

By creating matrices of proximal program objectives and matching methods and strategies to specific learning and change objectives, we can know (rather than guess) what one of these programs—the videotapes, the classes, the booklets—should include. Now, knowing what we want to change and how we want to bring about that change, we can let our creativity free to describe the program: the nature, scope, and sequence of the components of the intervention; what program materials are needed and what they would look like; and how the program will be implemented. Once some basic ideas are at hand, check back with representatives of each intervention group. What are their preferences and needs? At this preliminary stage, does the outlined program appear to be culturally competent?

Next, review existing materials. It may be tempting to do this at a much earlier stage in the process, but it is not until now that planners will have appropriate criteria with which to judge existing materials. Do they address the necessary learning and change objectives? Do they do so in a way that is likely to be successful given the determinant, the population, and the environment? Are the materials culturally competent for the intervention groups?

Writing Design Documents

If existing materials are not adequate and cannot be appropriately adapted or modified, the next step is to write design documents. These documents are the guides for program producers (writers, artists, videographers) as they create the actual program components. One must provide them with complete and accurate information on program parameters without doing their job for them. Certainly the design documents should detail the scope and sequence of the program, the materials that must be produced, the budget, timeline, and other constraints, and other information that must be considered both in the program producer's efforts and in the group's judging of those efforts. The earlier a program producer (for instance, the writer) can be brought into the planning process, the better. But at the very least, all the criteria and decisions the group has reached should be documented on paper and given to the program producers before they are asked for bids.

Pretesting Program Materials

The design documentation given to producers must specify that all materials must be pilot tested and revised in accordance with the results (National Cancer Institute, 1989). One need not—and should not—have a final, finished product to do pilot testing. Public service announcements can be presented in storyboard format. Booklets can be presented as text produced on a laser printer with sketches of the illustrations. Pilot testing should garner the most specific feedback possible, covering separate program elements as well as the program as a whole. For example, when pilot testing a newsletter that combines several strategies, such as role model stories, guided practice, and the presentation of information, we want to know the appeal and effect of each component, not just the appeal of the newsletter as a whole. Therefore, we might put a survey box at the end of each article or address each article separately in a focus group. After pilot testing, the information is summarized and changes are made. However, it is important to remember to refer back to the methods and strategies list and to the matrices when making changes in program elements. If elements that were designed to have a certain impact are dropped, they must be replaced with elements that are designed to have a similar effect.

Adoption and Implementation

The impact of a health education program will be determined not only by the demonstrated effectiveness of the intervention under test conditions, but also by the quality of program implementation and the proportion of the target population exposed to the program. To prevent the problem of inadequate diffusion of useful programs, planning must include additional interventions for influencing program adoption, implementation, and sustainability. This is the fourth step in Intervention Mapping. Powerful diffusion interventions are important because program adopters and implementers are most often not the program developers. For example, a disease management company may develop a program for use by managed care organizations. Even if representatives of those who deliver the program have been involved in program development, they may not feel "ownership" of the program or have the skills to implement it. Further, program implementation inevitably requires changes in both the program and the implementing organization; implementers must be prepared for the inevitable organizational disruption caused by any innovation (Ottoson and Green, 1987). Planning for adoption and implementation of a program begins in the first moments of program development when a team is organized. A linkage system is formed to include in the planning group those who will use or implement the program as well as representatives of the target group.

Writing Performance Objectives for Adoption and Implementation

The work of Rogers (1995) and others over several decades has laid the groundwork for how to get programs adopted, implemented, and continued over time. Often this is referred to as diffusion and focuses on program adoption and initial use. However, over the past decade, increasing attention has been given to the processes involved with both program implementation (Monahan and Scheirer, 1988; Roberts-Gray, 1985; Scheirer, 1994) and the continuation of programs (Goodman, Steckler, and Kegler, 1997; Shediac-Rizkallah and Bone, 1998). Diffusion is thought of as generally moving from awareness of a need or innovation, through decisions to adopt the innovation, to initial use and program continuation. The planner must think of what is required for each of these phases. The performance objectives for this step are similar to performance objectives in Step One specified for health-related behavior, except that the behaviors in Step Four are adoption, implementation, and (depending on goals selected for sustainability) either maintenance, institutionalization, or capacity building for sustaining health effects. The performance objectives provide the specificity for the program planners to make clear what performance will constitute use with acceptable fidelity and completeness.

Selecting Determinants for Adoption and Implementation

As with the performance objectives of health-related behaviors, the performance objectives for program use will have a set of hypothetical determinants (factors that are likely to influence their performance). The determinants may be personal (located within the individuals responsible for adoption and implementation) or external (social or structural factors that might serve as barriers or facilitators). The processes for selecting determinants are the same as those recommended for the determinants of health-related behavior. The starting activity is to brainstorm with the planning group (including the linkage system) on a list of factors that will facilitate or serve as barriers to accomplishing the performance objectives for each stage. To refine or add to this list, review the literature and the information from potential program users.

Preparing a Matrix for Adoption, Implementation, and Sustainability

A matrix of proximal adoption and implementation objectives is developed with adoption, implementation, and sustainability objectives juxtaposed to personal and external determinants. The synthesis of each objective with a determinant produces a proximal objective. These are then operationalized using methods and strategies to form a concrete, comprehensive, theory-based plan for adoption and implementation. In Table 4.4, sample performance objectives for adopting and implementing an asthma program that consists of physician training and use of an action plan are listed on the left side of the matrix and hypothetical personal determinants for adoption and implementation are listed along the top. A complete program matrix would also include performance objectives and determinants for maintenance and institutionalization and their corresponding hypothetical determinants.

Once we have specified learning and change objectives, we then develop methods and strategies to encourage adoption and implementation. The product for this task is a detailed plan for accomplishing program adoption and implementation by influencing the behavior of individuals or groups who will make decisions about using the program.

Using the Planning Process to Plan Evaluation

In the process of Intervention Mapping, planners make decisions about learning and change objectives, methods, strategies, and implementation. Although the decisions are based on theory, evidence from research, and knowledge of the at-risk and intervention groups, they still may not be optimal. Through monitoring and evaluation, Step Five of Intervention Mapping, planners can determine if decisions were correct at each mapping step.

Developing an Evaluation Model and Posing Questions

The first task is to build an evaluation model that includes the relations between the products of each Intervention Mapping step. To evaluate the effect of an intervention, evaluators pose questions regarding reduction of the health and social problems (outcomes), changes in behavior and environment (impact), and changes in

Table 4.4. Pediatric Asthma Matrix for Health Care Providers—Practice Adoption.

Performance Objectives	Outcome Expectations	Perception of Program Characteristics	Perceived Social Norms or Physician Characteristics	Knowledge
Adoption				
Seek information on program and acquire program	Belief that if asthma were managed better, children in practice would be healthier and standard of care better	Belief that program is simple, not costly, and "trialable"; has observable impact and scientific basis; fits with adopter's practice	Perception that valued colleagues with similar practices are using the program	Description of the program and how to order it
Ask office manager and nurse to review program				
Discuss program fit with staff		Belief that program will help asthma patients congruent with personal practice and quality standards		
Implementation				
Schedule asthma and suspected asthma visits with time to allow adequate exam and action plan review	Belief that slightly longer visits are required to better manage asthma to result in healthier children			
Review videotape on action plan use		Perception that program is simple but requires certain skills to use the action plan appropriately	Belief that colleagues would need added instruction to use action plan appropriately	Description of brief physician training as part of program
Use action plan as described on tape	Belief that action plan will result in asthma managed better, healthier children, and better standard of care	Belief that action plan is simple, fits with philosophy of patient-provider interaction, can be tried without great cost to practice, and will have observable results	Belief that physicians similar to self would use an action plan in the way described on video	Description of use of action plan as requiring understanding of family goals and so on

determinants of performance objectives (impact). All of these variables have been defined in a measurable way during the preceding steps. Health and quality-of-life variables and goals for change were defined in the needs assessment. Proposed changes in behavior and environment were specified in the first step of Intervention Mapping, as were performance objectives, determinants, and learning and change objectives. To describe process, evaluators pose questions regarding the implementation of methods, strategies, and program.

Using the Matrices As Measurement Blueprints

One of the ways that Intervention Mapping is most helpful to evaluation efforts is in the development of such measures as tests and questionnaires. Often when planners want to measure behavior, environment, or determinants, they need to measure constructs that are very specifically related to their program planning. For example, intended effects on intervening behavioral variables for health care providers in our asthma example are listed as performance objectives on the left side of the matrix in Table 4.2 on page 95. If we wanted to measure or observe behavior, we would begin to develop self-report or observational measures working from the performance objectives. If we are interested in measuring impact on determinants, the columns become the instrument blueprints for measures of behavioral capability, skills and self-efficacy, perceived social norms, and outcome expectations. The items within the matrix cells are the content of instrument items that must then be worded correctly for the measurement of the specific construct.

It must be noted that the process is not simple. Each construct will have a literature regarding its measurement and the planner should be familiar with it. For instance, self-efficacy items would be constructed in terms of confidence for performing specific behavior, and the planner would want to read the literature on the measurement of self-efficacy for guidance on how to construct the items and the scale (see, for example, Bartholomew, Parcel, Swank, and

Czyzewski, 1993). Once items are developed and instruments prepared, they should be subject to pilot testing and investigations of reliability and validity.

Conclusion

Even though we present Intervention Mapping as a series of steps, the process is intended to be practiced as an iterative rather than as a completely linear process. Program developers move back and forth between tasks and steps as they gain information and perspective from various activities, tasks, or steps. However, the process is also cumulative. The developer bases each step on the previous steps, and inattention to a step can jeopardize the potential effectiveness of the intervention by narrowing the scope and compromising the validity with which later steps are conducted. Sometimes planners may be carried away by momentum in the process of the planning group or, alternatively, may be overwhelmed and bypass a step. Fortunately, most of the time one can backtrack and include, repeat, or elaborate on a neglected step.

A Focus on Changing Behavior Through Determinant Change

Using the PRECEDE model as a needs assessment tool helps the planner begin to focus on behavior and environment rather than on intervention content as a basis for program planning. PRECEDE is a valuable tool for justifying programs with epidemiological analyses, documenting outcomes in terms of health and quality of life, and linking both the health and social problems to behavior and environment.

Intervention Mapping can take the disease management field to the next level of planning, which is to focus on changing determinants in order to change behavior and its context. Moving from the all-too-common explanation of "They don't know anything about [the disease]" to a comprehensive picture of why a certain behavior is or is not performed has the potential of enabling powerful interventions. The Intervention Mapping matrices can be a key to this process.

The process of changing behavior is at best complex and at worst a black box of unknowns. As the tools of PRECEDE and Intervention Mapping are transferred from health education to disease management, they can contribute a systematic process for managing that complexity and for hypothesizing and testing, through intervention evaluation, what is in the black box for any particular disease management issue.

Enhancing Creativity

Intervention Mapping can also enable planners to creatively produce feasible programs that have a high likelihood of being effective. Good program planning not only provides the basis for creative program planning, but also provides the vehicles for communicating program specifications to ad agencies and production specialists such as writers and artists. The better the planning at the beginning of a project, the more creative the developmental and production process can be, while at the same time enhancing the intervention's deliverability and the likelihood of its producing the desired outcomes. Thus, the Intervention Map provides a guide for everyone involved in the planning process to travel a common path from start to finish of program planning and development.

References

Bandura, A. *Social Foundation of Thought and Action: A Social Cognitive Theory.* Englewood Cliffs, N.J.: Prentice Hall, 1986.

Bartholomew, L. K., Parcel, G. S., and Kok, G. "Intervention Mapping: A Process for Designing Theory- and Data-Based Health Education Programs." *Health Education and Behavior,* 1998, 25(5), 545–563.

Bartholomew, L. K., Parcel, G. S., Kok, G., and Gottlieb, N. *Intervention Mapping: A Process for Designing Theory- and Evidence-Based Health Education Programs.* Mountain View, Calif.: Mayfield Publishing, 2000.

Bartholomew, L. K., Parcel, G. S., Swank, P. R., and Czyzewski, D. I. "Measuring Self-Efficacy Expectations for the Self-Management of Cystic Fibrosis." *Chest,* 1993, 103(5), 1524–1530.

Bartholomew, L. K., and others. "Development of an Education Program to Promote the Self-Management of Cystic Fibrosis: Application of a Diagnostic Framework." *Health Education Quarterly*, 1991, 18(4), 429–443.

Bartholomew, L. K., and others. "Performance Objectives for the Self-Management of Cystic Fibrosis." *Patient Education and Counseling*, 1993, 22(1), 15–25.

Bartholomew, L. K., and others. "Watch, Discover, Think, and Act: A Model for Patient Education Program Development." *Patient Education and Counseling*, 2000, 39(2–3), 253–268.

Basch, C. E. "Focus Group Interview: An Underutilized Research Technique for Improving Theory and Practice in Health Education." *Health Education Quarterly*, 1987, 14, 411–448.

Bauman, L. J., and Adair, E. G. "The Use of Ethnographic Interviewing to Inform Questionnaire Construction." *Health Education Quarterly*, 1992, 19, 9–23.

Becker, M. H. "The Health Belief Model and Sick Role Behavior." *Health Education Monographs*, 1974, 2, 409–419.

Clark, N. M., and Zimmerman, B. J. "A Social Cognitive View of Self-Regulated Learning About Health." *Health Education Research*, 1990, 5, 371–379.

Cullen, K. W., Bartholomew, L. K., Parcel, G. S., and Kok, G. "Intervention Mapping: Use of Theory and Data in the Development of a Fruit and Vegetable Nutrition Program for Girl Scouts." *Journal of Nutrition Education*, 1998, 30(4), 188–195.

Dawson, K. P., and others. "An Evaluation of the Action Plans of Children with Asthma." *Journal of Paediatrics and Child Health*, 1995, 31(1), 21–23.

Expert Panel Report 2: Guidelines for the Diagnosis and Management of Asthma. National Asthma Education and Prevention Program, Clinical Practice Guidelines. NIH publication no. 97-4051, July 1997. Bethesda, Md.: National Institutes of Health, National Heart, Lung, and Blood Institute, 1997.

Finkelstein, J. A., and others. "Quality of Care for Preschool Children with Asthma: The Role of Social Factors and Practice Setting." *Pediatrics*, 1995, 95(3), 389–394.

Gilmore, G. D., Campbell, M. D., and Becker, B. L. *Needs Assessment Strategies for Health Education and Health Promotion.* Indianapolis, Ind.: Benchmark Press, 1989.

Glanz, K., Lewis, F. M., and Rimer, B. K. (eds.). *Health Behavior and Health Education: Theory, Research, and Practice.* (2nd ed.) San Francisco: Jossey-Bass, 1997.

Glasgow, R. W., McCaul, K. D., and Schafer, L. C. "Barriers to Regimen Adherence Among Persons with Insulin-Dependent Diabetes." *Journal of Behavioral Medicine*, 1986, 9(1), 65–77.

Goodman, R. M., Steckler, A., and Kegler, M. C. "Mobilizing Organizations for Health Enhancement: Theories of Organizational Change." In K. Glanz, F. M. Lewis, and B. K. Rimer (eds.), *Health Behavior and Health Education: Theory, Research, and Practice.* (2nd ed.) San Francisco: Jossey-Bass, 1997, pp. 287–312.

Green, L. W., and Kreuter, M. W. *Health Promotion Planning: An Educational and Ecological Approach.* (3rd ed.) Mountain View, Calif.: Mayfield Publishing, 1999.

Homer, C. J., and others. "Does Quality of Care Affect Rates of Hospitalization for Childhood Asthma?" *Pediatrics*, 1996, 98(1), 18–23.

Janz, N. K., and Becker, M. H. "The Health Belief Model: A Decade Later." *Health Education Quarterly*, 1984, 11(1), 1–47.

Kok, G., and others. "Social Psychology and Health Education." In W. Stroebe and M. Hewstone (eds.), *European Review of Social Psychology.* Chichester, U.K.: Wiley, 1996, pp. 241–282.

Kreuger, R. A. *Focus Groups: A Practical Guide for Applied Research.* Newbury Park, Calif.: Sage, 1988.

Lazarus, R., and Folkman, S. *Stress, Appraisal and Coping.* New York: Springer, 1984.

Lieu, T. A., and others. "Outpatient Management Practices Associated with Reduced Risk of Pediatric Asthma Hospitalization and Emergency Department Visits." *Pediatrics*, 1997, 100(3 pt 1), 334–341.

Maibach, E., and Parrot, R. L. (eds.). *Designing Health Messages: Approaches from Communication Theory and Public Health Practice.* Thousand Oaks, Calif.: Sage, 1995.

McLeroy, K. R., Bibeau, D., Steckler, A., and Glanz, K. "An Ecological Perspective on Health Promotion Programs." *Health Education Quarterly*, 1988, 15(4), 351–377.

McLeroy, K. R., and others. "Social Science Theory in Health Education: Time for a New Model?" [editorial] *Health Education Research*, 1995, 8(3), 305–312.

Minkler, M. (ed.). *Community Organizing and Community Building for Health.* New Brunswick, N.J.: Rutgers University Press, 1997.

Monahan, J. L., and Scheirer, M. A. "The Role of Linking Agents in the Diffusion of Health Promotion Programs." *Health Education Quarterly*, 1988, 15(4), 417–433.

Murray, N., Kelder, S., Parcel, G., and Orpinas, P. "Development of an Intervention Map for a Parent Education Intervention to Prevent Violence Among Hispanic Middle School Students." *Journal of School Health*, 1998, 68(2), 46–52.

National Cancer Institute. *Making Health Communication Programs Work: A Planner's Guide*. Publication no. 89-1493. Bethesda, Md.: National Institutes of Health, 1989.

Ottoson, J. M., and Green, L. W. "Reconciling Concept and Context: Theory of Implementation." In W. B. Ward and M. H. Becker (eds.), *Advances in Health Education and Promotion, 2*. Greenwich, Conn.: JAI Press, 1987, pp. 353–382.

Richard, L., and others. "Assessment of the Integration of the Ecological Approach in Health Promotion Programs." *American Journal of Health Promotion*, 1996, 10(4), 318–328.

Roberts-Gray, C. "Managing the Implementation of Innovations." *Education and Program Planning*, 1985, 8, 261–269.

Robertson, A., and Minkler, M. "New Health Promotion Movement: A Critical Examination." *Health Education Quarterly*, 1994, 21(3), 295–312.

Rogers, E. M. *Diffusion of Innovations* (4th ed.). New York: Free Press, 1995.

Ruiter, R., Kok, G., and Abraham, C. *Fear Appeals in Health Education: Theory and Research*. Internal report. Maastricht, the Netherlands: Department of Health Education, Universiteit Maastricht, 1999.

Scheirer, M. A. "Designing and Using Process Evaluation." In J. S. Wholey, H. P. Hatry, and K. E. Newcomer (eds.), *Handbook of Practical Program Evaluation*. San Francisco: Jossey-Bass, 1994, pp. 40–68.

Shediac-Rizkallah, M. C., and Bone, L. R. "Planning for the Sustainability of Community-Based Health Programs: Conceptual Frameworks and Future Directions for Research, Practice and Policy." *Health Education Research: Theory and Practice*, 1998, 13(1), 87–108.

Simons-Morton, D. G., Simons-Morton, B. G., Parcel, G. S., and Bunker, J. F. "Influencing Personal and Environmental Conditions for Community Health: A Multilevel Intervention Model." *Family and Community Health*, 1988, 11(2), 25–35.

Skinner, C. S., Strecher, V. J., and Hospers, H. "Physicians' Recommendations for Mammography: Do Tailored Messages Make a Difference?" *American Journal of Public Health*, 1994, 84(1), 43–49.

Sockrider, M. M., and others. "Pilot Evaluation of the Children's Asthma Center Consultative Clinic: Family Outcomes at 1 Year after Initial Visit."

Unpublished report to the administrative committee of the Children's Asthma Center, Texas Children's Hospital, Houston, 1998.

Soriano, F. I. *Conducting Needs Assessments: A Multidisciplinary Approach.* Thousand Oaks, Calif.: Sage, 1995.

Stokols, D. "Translating Social Ecological Theory into Guidelines for Community Health Promotion." *American Journal of Health Promotion,* 1996, 10(4), 282–298.

Strecher, V. J., and others. "The Effects of Computer-Tailored Smoking Cessation Messages in Family Practice Settings." *Journal of Family Practice,* Sept. 1994, 39(3), 262–270.

Tortolero, S. R., and others. "Estimates of Asthma Prevalence in Sixty Southeast Texas Inner-City Schools." Manuscript in preparation.

Tyrrell, S., and others. "A Program to Improve the Asthma-Related Environment of Urban Elementary Schools: An Application of the Intervention Mapping Framework." Manuscript in preparation.

Veen, P. *Sociale Psychologie Toegepast: Van Probleem naar Oplossing.* [Applying Social Psychology: From Problem to Solution.] Alphen aan den Rijn, Netherlands: Samson, 1985.

Witkin, B. R., and Altschuld, J. W. *Planning and Conducting Needs Assessments.* Thousand Oaks, Calif.: Sage, 1995.

5

Using Telephone-Based Interventions

Terry Mason

Shortly after the invention of the telephone, a pioneering physician probably called a patient to see how she was feeling—and inexorably tied the telephone to the American health care delivery system!

The telephone has become one of the most widely used means of communication in the health care field. Depending on the specialty, between 10 to 57 percent of patient contacts are by phone (Friedman and others, 1996). Not only do hundreds of thousands of health care professionals now talk with patients by phone every day, the past ten to twenty years have seen widespread growth in other therapeutic uses of the telephone.

A Brief History

Two ventures helped the health care industry begin to explore new uses for the telephone in medicine. "Ask-a-Nurse" lines, developed in the 1980s to both improve patient access to care and market hospital and clinic services, were one of the first telephone-based interventions to be incorporated into health care delivery systems. These programs often linked to libraries of prerecorded health messages that allowed patients to access general medical information quickly and conveniently. Both of these programs were particularly helpful in serving geographically dispersed populations.

By the mid-1980s, health professionals were using a larger variety of innovative telephone-based interventions to improve patient care and cut the cost of service delivery. Telephone programs were designed to answer patient questions about medicines and help people understand how to use health care services more wisely and make more informed decisions about health care (Hallam, 1989). At the same time, providers began experimenting with the telephone as a modality for delivering interventions in disease prevention, high-risk and demand management, and disease management.

The establishment of criteria for identification of target populations combined with the increased ability to access databases to identify potential participants for intervention programs encouraged the growth of outbound calling programs. Outbound phone programs are convenient, confidential, and increase the range of potential applications of telephone interventions (Mason, 1995; Soet, 1997; Balas and others, 1997; Friedman and others, 1996; "Phone Counseling," 1995). Calls can be made to collect data, remind patients about follow-up, check on patient progress, provide lifestyle and emotional counseling, and assist decision making.

Initially, outbound telephone intervention services were primarily marketed to employers. Corporations would buy the service to reach high-risk and high-demand employees, targeting the individuals who spend the greatest share of health care dollars for special interventions. Once criteria were established to identify people with elevated health risks or who used a high volume of health care services, outbound phone calls could be initiated to reach these target populations. Because the earlier ventures relied on the patient calling the provider to request a service, outbound programs represented a major conceptual change in telephone-based intervention.

Increased linkage with claims and patient data systems has increased the ways the telephone can be used in health care. The telephone is now used for monitoring, improving compliance, counseling, enhancing patient decision making, and managing risks and disease.

Telephonic interventions may also help reduce health services utilization and health costs. For example, managed care organizations (MCOs) are actively developing systems that integrate clinical records and claims experience. Using a telephone-based intervention system, a population can be identified and tracked over time; the same system can simultaneously measure the overall effectiveness of the intervention.

The past twenty years' experience with telephone interventions has improved our understanding of the use of both inbound and outbound calling strategies. Telephonic interventions reached approximately thirteen million contracted lives in 1994 ("Phone Counseling," 1995). To date, insurance carriers have been slow to reimburse for these types of programs, but government agencies are warming to the idea. A few states are beginning to mandate insurance payment for telephonic medical care.

A Brief Summary of the Research

A MEDLINE search was conducted for the past ten years using the word "telephone" in the search criteria and another search turned up 147 citations in journals from the United States, England, Canada, Japan, Israel, and Australia. Approximately 25 percent of the articles found by these studies were researched for this chapter. This review of the literature reveals that telephone-based intervention programs have most commonly been studied using the following methods:

- Comparison of phone use to print use

- Comparison of phone calls to clinic visits

- Comparison of in-person surveys to phone surveys

- Comparison of print reminders to phone reminders

- Comparison of use of print alone and phone alone to print and phone together

- Comparison of phone use across interventions that use multiple modalities

- Reports of individual interventions that use the telephone to deliver services

Telephone use is reported on for:

- Employed populations

- Free-ranging community populations (that is, not grouped by geography, employment, health care provider, or other characteristic)

- Rural populations

- Inner-city populations and homeless populations

- Women

- The elderly

- People with a single chronic disease or multiple ones or lifestyle risks

Telephone use is also studied in the delivery of the following types of interventions:

- Marketing of hospital and clinic services

- Demand management

- High-risk management

- Patient reminder calls

- Behavioral and psychological counseling

- Compliance enhancement

- Survey questionnaires

- Patient triage

Because most of the research published to date examines a single intervention, it offers little help in defining when telephone programs will be most effective or efficient. Replication of results is scarce and cost effectiveness is only examined in a few single interventions.

Although meta-analysis is rare (only two were found), we can observe these trends in the literature:

- Outbound calling programs reach and enroll larger percentages of targeted populations than other modalities such as group programs or one-on-one counseling at a fitness center, clinic, or physician's office.

- Participation in older model, call-in type employee assistance services or Ask-a-Pharmacist or Ask-a-Nurse lines can range from approximately 5 to 30 percent of eligible employees in a given year ("Phone Counseling," 1995); in that same period, new outbound calling model programs can reach as much as 70 percent of the targeted population (Balas and others, 1997; Sleek, 1997). This increase in participation levels strengthens intervention results (Friedman and others, 1996; Wasson and others, 1992; Davis and others, 1987).

Dropout for telephone-based intervention programs is very low—frequently less than 10 percent. In comparison, the dropout rate for group programs held at the worksite can run as high as 60 percent (King and others, 1994; Soet, 1997; O'Donnell, 1996). More than 90 percent of Americans work in companies with fewer than one hundred employees. Most face-to-face and print- or video-based prevention and health promotion programs were developed for large worksites, and most of the scientific studies documenting behavioral and economic changes have been based on experience at large worksites (O'Donnell, 1996). Unfortunately, on-site delivery models developed for large worksites do not always transfer well to small sites—but telephonic solutions (especially when combined with print materials) do appear to respond to the needs of smaller or more dispersed populations (O'Donnell, 1996; Mason, 1996).

Access to routine care is problematic in most rural and some inner-city populations. States with dispersed or hard-to-reach populations can now opt for telemedicine solutions to help address access issues. In Maine, six rural towns developed a program that funneled all primary care through nurses. The nurses used both outbound and inbound calls to facilitate access to the right service. Nurses also provided information on care and prevention ("Phone Counseling," 1995; Anders, 1997).

Triage systems primarily rely on phone and print modalities. About thirty-five million Americans currently have access to phone triage systems (Anders, 1997). In one large company, 40 percent of patients who call the triage lines are not sent to physicians at all. Only 2 percent are sent to the emergency room and 15 percent are sent to urgent care. The rest are sent to see a health professional for consultation (Anders, 1997). Triage systems are a powerful way to address access issues, hard-to-reach populations, and difficult patient follow-up scenarios.

People like the phone modality. Patient and participant satisfaction have been high across the different types of telephone-based programming ("Phone Counseling," 1995; "Patients More Apt to Admit Mental Disorders," 1997; Friedman and others, 1996; Siegel and others, 1988; Curry and others, 1995; Zhu and others, 1996).

Surveys by phone often yield better results than survey questions asked face to face.

Studies are increasingly showing that surveys done by interactive voice response systems are very effective, increase consistency of data collection, and are well liked by participants (Friedman and others, 1996; Siegel and others, 1988). This has been particularly true for surveys designed to help clinicians diagnose mental illnesses ("Patients More Apt to Admit Mental Disorders," 1997).

Phone-based programs compare favorably to print-based programs. Phone works better than print alone or print with one or two phone calls for behavioral changes (Davis and others, 1987; Balas and others, 1997). Telephone reminder calls also work better than print reminders for compliance (Wasson and others, 1992). Self-report by phone is as valid as self-report in other modalities, including print and face to face (Soet, 1997).

Multiple telephone sessions for counseling interventions work better than single sessions (Balas and others, 1997; Curry and others, 1995). Behavioral change results by phone are comparable with behavioral change programs in any other modality (for similar numbers of sessions) (Curry and others, 1995; Zhu and others, 1996; Soet, 1997). For smoking, telephone-based program results are not improved, but are comparable. Smoking cessation results appear to be constant across modalities: a 30 percent quit rate at the end of one year (Curry and others, 1995; Zhu and others, 1996). Phone-based interventions can be less expensive than in-person, face-to-face modalities (Zhu and others, 1996; Soet, 1997).

Phone-based chronic disease management programs have comparable results with group programs with a much lower dropout rate. Group program dropout ranges between 40 and 60 percent, whereas phone program dropout is generally less than 10 percent. This may indicate that overall results are better with the phone intervention because reach and capture statistics are better (Zhu and others, 1996).

The telephone is a less conspicuous program delivery option. Some areas of medical care, like social work and mental health, may still carry stigmas. When this is the case, the telephone helps people access services while maintaining confidentiality and personal privacy. The mental health field has been actively exploring the use of the telephone. In a study of the computerized version of the diagnostic tool Primary Care Evaluation Disorders (PRIME MD), comparisons were made between clinician-administered and phone-administered survey instruments designed to improve physicians' ability to detect psychiatric disorders in patients with medical complaints. In this study, respondents were twice as likely to admit alcohol abuse on the phone, and the phone-administered surveys were three times as likely to detect obsessive-compulsive disorder. Panic disorders, for some unknown reason, were detected twice as often by the physicians ("Patients More Apt to Admit Mental Disorders," 1997).

Another study, looking at mild depression treated by family practitioners by phone, reported decreased depression and improved functioning after short telephone sessions with the physician (Lynch, Tamburrino, and Nagel, 1997). The American Psychological Association has been actively looking into product development, policy, marketing, and access issues of providing therapy by phone and with video monitoring (Sleek, 1997).

These trends in the literature indicate that the telephone is a successful intervention modality, and studies on specific intervention types are most promising. The studies give us information we need to design effective and efficient interventions. We are beginning to tease out which types of intervention, singly and in combination, will be the most effective.

To use the telephone effectively, it is important to understand the range of technologies and modalities available today. Some of the most promising include voice mailbox, patient callback and reminder programs, menu-based prerecorded messages, and interactive voice response systems.

Voice Mailbox

Voice mailboxes are common in clinic practices; what is exciting are the newer ways that this technology is being used. Connections between computer databases and answering machines are becoming easier to program and operate, which means that data captured by voice mail can automatically be downloaded from the phone to the computer.

Patient reporting is one of the newer uses of the voice mailbox. This application is excellent for monitoring home care and chronic disease. Voice mailboxes can also be used in weight management and dietary recall programs or for any behavioral intervention that calls for consistent practice and monitoring. Such monitoring has been shown to increase adherence, improve the patient-provider relationship, and increase patient satisfaction (Friedman and others, 1996; Siegel and others, 1988; Wasson and others, 1992; Balas and others, 1997).

Patient Callback and Reminder Programs

Since the 1970s studies have shown positive outcomes for patient callback and reminder programs. Consistency for regular appointments (teeth cleaning, mammograms, gynecological screening) is improved with reminders. Software for scheduling provides operators with dates and patient names and telephone numbers. Research consistently shows that phone reminders work better than print reminders. The combination of the two currently appears to be most effective (Wasson and others, 1992; Davis and others, 1987; Balas and others, 1997).

One of the newer applications links reminder calls with counseling on the need for follow-up. Reminder calls plus counseling appear to work best with patients who, for various reasons, may not want to return to the clinic (Davis and others, 1987; King and others, 1994; Miller and others, 1989). The combination improves adherence and patient satisfaction, particularly when lack of access, anticipated pain, cost, and denial exist. In one study in a large managed care organization, counseling tripled the odds that a woman would have a mammogram (King and others, 1994). This intervention has also been done at other sites (Davis and others, 1987).

Menu-Based Prerecorded Messages

Prerecorded messages are selected from a menu by pushing a key on a touch-tone phone. For example, patients who call in may be asked to "Press 6 for a message on gum disease." The patient then receives a three- to five-minute message with general information about the topic.

Branching within prerecorded scripts for further tailoring is a fairly straightforward programming task that enhances the use of prerecorded messages by providing more personalized messages. For instance, smokers might be asked about whether or not they have set a quit date. If they have, the recording gives positive reinforcement; if they have not, the recording branches to provide more information about setting a date. Depth of branching is limited by the participant comfort level with the length of the phone call— usually about ten minutes.

Prerecorded messages can now provide much more than information; they can also assist in data collection and patient monitoring. In diabetes management programs, for instance, patients may use a prerecorded message program to report blood glucose monitoring results on a regular basis. The patient calls the number, accesses an account with a password, and enters responses to prerecorded questions. In a high-cholesterol management program, participants can take part in health-risk appraisal by using the same technology. Results are summarized at the end of the call and a printed report may be sent to the participant. These applications illustrate ways that the uses of prerecorded messages are currently being enhanced and expanded.

Interactive Voice Response

Interactive voice response systems are being developed and tested in health care settings, although this methodology has been used extensively in other fields, particularly for marketing and political surveys. This telephone intervention technology is most promising because the medium can be tailored to the individual through software branching. The medium also helps control for differences in approach across counselors.

In the interactive voice response modality, a prerecorded tape with instructions leads participants through a survey or educational program. Participants can respond verbally or by pushing a key on a touch-tone key pad. The responses given by the participants are captured by the system; data thus collected can then be used to guide follow-up and to provide outcome measurement.

Lower blood pressure and increased adherence were found in one study measuring the effectiveness of interactive voice response. The study compared usual care with usual care plus telephone monitoring. The average age of most of the participants in this study was seventy-six, and the participants were mostly from urban settings. Acceptance of the interactive voice response was very high and there were positive outcomes in health status (Friedman and others, 1996).

Interactive voice response programs have the least research and the most promise of all contemporary phone intervention modalities. Currently, the best results appear to be for interactive voice response systems that monitor and track. The literature shows that participants find the computer voice programs easy to use and understand and that the programs motivate them to make changes. Published results are most positive for monitoring and assessment programming. There is less evidence that these programs work as well in behaviorally based interventions.

The technology now exists to make a wider range of interactive voice response programming possible, but our experience with outcomes, cost, and satisfaction is neither consistent nor widely published. At this time, we are also lacking a cost-benefit analysis for this particular technology. As the technology becomes less expensive, however, and results more available, we fully expect interactive voice response intervention systems to become a major growth area.

Mixed Modality Interventions

We have learned from marketing research that a message is better heard when repeated in different ways. And we have learned from adult education research that adults vary in the way they learn best. Including telephone delivery in an intervention modality mix should, therefore, increase both marketing and learning opportunities. However, although the telephone has increasingly been included in mixed modality interventions, to date there have been few reports that have looked across studies to assess how well the telephone is doing in these mixes.

Very few interventions rely on a single modality. Phone, print, screenings, posters, media messages, and group programs are used together to maximize effect and participation. Often the phone will be linked with print and screenings for disease management and risk management programs. What seems clear is that the power of the telephone is immeasurably increased when linked to other modalities like patient services and screenings, group programs, and personalized print materials.

In one meta-analysis, results were reported on the efficacy of distance-medicine technologies in clinical practice and health care outcomes in eighty clinical trials. The studies reviewed used computerized communication or telephone reminders or both, telephone follow-up and counseling, interactive telephone systems, after-hours telephone access, and telephone screening. Sixty-three percent of the studies reported positive outcomes, improved performance, or other significant benefits. Findings included greater continuity of care, improved access, and supporting communication between physicians and patients (Balas and others, 1997).

Studies evaluating the use of the telephone for mammography, follow-up for abnormal pap smears, smoking programs, and management of lupus, asthma, and other chronic diseases have also been published, each reporting positive results when mixing the telephone with print, group, and in-person modalities. Behavioral interventions and patient reminder programs have compared print only with print and one phone call and with multiple phone calls and print. In these studies, the multiple phone calls with print interventions have been reported as significantly more effective (Balas and others, 1997; Curry and others, 1995; Zhu and others, 1996; Soet, 1997).

To increase overall effectiveness, the power and limitations of any one modality must be understood by the program designers. Print materials (such as flyers, posters, and news articles) reinforce messages, provide information, and promote other health-related activities. When the role of print is to market or reinforce, then succinct messages work best. When the role of print is to inform, then tailored information specific to the participant works best. Unless print materials are personalized, readership will often only reach 10 percent. With personalization, readership can be 60 percent or higher.

Combinations of print and phone will work best when the strengths and weaknesses of each are understood. Print and phone should reinforce each other in both timing and content. Print can be used to market and inform; the telephone can be used to educate and counsel. For instance, if a behavioral intervention is marketed through print correspondence, program enrollment could be by phone. Alternatively, the intervention could be delivered by phone and print materials could be used to supply additional content information during the program or as a follow-up to help prevent recidivism. The task of the program designer is to understand each modality and the relationships between the modalities to create the strongest intervention.

Telephone compliance programs are most effective when delivered to participants who have recently been prescribed a medical treatment (Davis and others, 1987; King and others, 1994; Rimer and others, 1994; Miller and others, 1989). Assessments to identify barriers to adherence also help in compliance programming. An empowering model seems to work best using the same counselor over time to build rapport and trust. The availability of good assessment, results-oriented intervention, and personal touch seem to yield the best results (Davis and others, 1987; Zhu and others, 1996; Rimer and others, 1994).

Combining screening with phone intervention programs is very common. Screenings are often used to identify potential participants. The screening heightens health awareness and acts as an enrollment opportunity for further follow-up programming. Experience has shown that participation in follow-up programming is enhanced if participants hear about these programs at the screening. Follow-up programming should also be scheduled to start as soon as possible after the screening to capitalize on the increased health awareness of participants.

Increasing peer support through group phone programs (party lines), e-mail, and message boards have thus far been limited because many people do not have access to this technology. More than 50 percent of the United States population is currently on-line. That number is projected to grow quickly (McConneaughey, Nila, and Sloan, 1995). There are already tens of thousands of health programs on-line that offer access to the latest research, chat rooms, and bulletin boards. What effect these media will have on the health care industry is unknown, but as access grows so will effect—and the opportunities for using the computer, modem, and phone for intervention will continue to expand.

We need more research to help us understand the power of the telephone alone and the telephone in conjunction with other modalities. The next decade should reveal better ways to unlock the potential of the telephone in health care delivery and prevention and management of disease.

Specific Types of Interventions

Although the literature on exactly why telephone-based interventions are effective is slim, we do have sufficient experience to make some observations about the most effective ways to use the telephone in behaviorally based programs; with high-risk, high-demand employee populations; and in the marketing of health interventions.

Behavioral Interventions

The delivery of behavioral change programs by phone began to emerge in the late 1980s and has become increasingly more sophisticated and cost effective (Soet, 1997). Early models transferred the inpatient counseling model to the phone. This meant counselors spent between twenty and sixty minutes on phone calls, making this a relatively expensive intervention technique. More recently developed programs featuring targeted assessments and short-term counseling models have cut counselors' time on the phone without losing effectiveness. Some programs offer good results with an average of ten minutes per call (Friedman and others, 1996).

Seventy-five percent of participants in reported single-intervention programs (lupus, cardiovascular disease, asthma, diabetes, and hypertension, among others) self-report high satisfaction, being motivated to make change, and being able to name specific changes in their targeted area for behavioral change programming offered by phone (Soet, 1997; Friedman and others, 1996; Anders, 1997; Hallam, 1989). We do not yet have enough information to know whether the claims we see in these telephonic behavioral change programs will transfer to other topics or other behavior. However, because over half of the research studies published within the past three years describe telephone interventions with behavioral change components and outcome measures, we may soon have more explicit direction on what aspects of these programs are most effective.

In the meantime, it appears that behavioral programs with strong assessments to guide tailoring will be the most effective: the more straightforward the intervention, the better the results. Inconsistency across health counselors over time appears to be the biggest hurdle to consistent results. The differences in skill, educational background, personal style, and training of counselors affect the results of the program. Better training, increased use of specific assessments, computer-guided recordkeeping, intervention guidelines, and quality assurance standards have improved outcomes (Soet, 1997). As the programmatic software guidance systems become more user friendly and complete, so should consistent outcome measures.

High-Risk and High-Demand Employee Interventions

An increased ability to identify and target populations with specific risks, diagnoses, and health service use patterns increases our opportunities for intervention, resulting in considerable growth in disease management, risk management, demand management, and patient decision-making programs. Models for these interventions use the telephone to deliver most of the intervention.

A high-risk patient may not necessarily be a high-demand patient or vice versa. The person with a chronic disease may be well-informed, competent, and assertive. It is likely, however, that most people will have more than one eligibility characteristic for these separate interventions. So although these programs have traditionally been marketed separately, newer models use the thinking behind all of them in one combined intervention ("Phone Counseling," 1995; Balas and others, 1997; Soet, 1997).

It makes sense to combine key elements to yield the best outcomes. Successful programs have good assessments, straightforward interventions, and measurable outcomes. The first step is to identify the individual who meets the eligibility requirements. Assessments then allow for tailoring of the interventions. The better the tailoring, the better the health and cost outcome measures (Rimer and others, 1994).

Marketing Health Interventions by Phone

When hospitals began marketing services through Ask-a-Nurse lines more than twenty years ago, those early programs were really more about marketing than improving access. However, while other business sectors have begun to rely primarily on targeted phone marketing, the health care sector has wisely chosen a more judicious approach.

People often do not like phone market attempts; calls often come during dinner hours and early on weekend mornings when most people are at home. When patient satisfaction is important to maintain membership, it is wise to choose marketing methods that do not alienate the patient.

Telephone marketing can work well, however, when the task is to target special populations for specific programming (Soet, 1997; King and others, 1994; Anders, 1997). For instance, a Pennsylvania

MCO calls smokers referred by primary care physicians to enroll them in a stop smoking program; a Massachusetts MCO does the same with patients identified as smokers from patient records. This strategy works best when the patient has some forewarning that the call is coming. Newsletters announcing the program, targeted mailings, posters, information flyers left in clinic waiting rooms, and physician involvement in recruitment seem to soften the marketing edge and build acceptance for the calls.

Achieving good enrollment numbers is not an educational effort; it is a marketing effort. The message must capture and engage the person in the program and the timing must be right to maximize results.

Calls made within a few weeks of diagnosis, screening, or physician recommendation may yield a 70 percent sign-up (Soet, 1997; King and others, 1994; Miller and others, 1989). The greater the distance between first patient contact and enrollment call, the smaller the yield will be. Enrollment figures can drop to 30 percent when the marketing call is made after three months from first contact (Mason, 1996). This is still better than the yield from open sign-up for on-site programming. Two different outreach programs have shown that approximately 70 percent of a targeted contact list can be reached with two phone calls and that additional phone calls may not be cost effective.

Telephone marketing interventions may be delivered by in-house staff or by outside experts. For example, professional marketing services can be contracted to make scripted enrollment calls on behalf of a health care facility. This industry has technology in place, trained staff, and reporting capabilities and their expertise on what works can be helpful. Professional services can be particularly useful when the number of persons to be contacted is very large. On the other hand, smaller target populations may be reached more easily and cost effectively by office staff. Staff are more familiar with the services and can answer more questions.

Growth of Telephone Interventions in Hospital and Clinic Settings

In the past twenty years, hospitals have moved toward patient-focused care and case management models that use critical care pathways to improve outcomes and patient satisfaction and cut costs.

Critical care pathways and case management work synergistically. Case managers use a systems approach to examine patient needs, coordinate care, and control costs. The critical care pathway also allows hospital personnel to help ensure that patients with similar problems and treatment plans have similar outcomes. A standardized course of treatment and a standardized method for analyzing patient deviations from expected outcomes facilitate decision making within the hospital.

As hospitals began to use these innovations with greater frequency, they also became more sophisticated in claims analysis, improving the linkages between cost (medical claims analysis) and care (patient experience and records) databases. The ability to target individuals by both patient experience and patient claims increased the opportunities for disease management programming. These hospital-based innovations are now widely accepted and are facilitating the use of the telephone in follow-up programming (Balas and others, 1997; Mason, 1995).

Some National Committee for Quality Assurance (NCQA) standards have also improved the climate for the development of telephone-based disease management programs. Specifically, the NCQA requires that members with chronic conditions be followed and assisted in managing their conditions. Similarly, the Health Plan Employer Data and Information Set, a measurement program offered by the NCQA, allows employer groups and consumers to compare performance of MCOs. They are compared on the basis of improvement in patient functional status, their follow-up and prevention programs, and whether they take an active role in managing chronic disease.

However, if managed care organizations only treat patients when they present for care, they may be limited to treating patients with acute care needs. And if MCOs only offer follow-up and prevention programs on-site, they may reach only 5 to 30 percent of their target population. So it makes sense that we are increasingly seeing models of disease management that use the telephone as part of an ongoing, population-based intervention strategy.

Increased regulation, innovations in hospital care, quality assurance measures, improved access to data, and nurse call lines have helped hospitals and MCOs understand the growing importance of disease management as part of a population-based strategy. The telephone has become an increasingly important modality as the health care community struggles with reaching dispersed populations for continuity-of-care programs. As our access to, and comfort with, technology improves and as the cost goes down, we will undoubtedly see more and more applications involving the telephone as an integral part of health care delivery.

Conclusion

Software guidance systems are critical in managing phone programming. A good software system allows program managers to achieve quality assurance standards across each program component, control for consistency across phone operators, and allow for outcome measures in health and cost.

Linking with aligned databases is critical for identifying potential participants and maximizing outcomes in care. Linkage between program modalities is needed to correctly assess the power of each separate modality. Software management systems that allow for linked databases are still problematic, however. Their development will be necessary to both manage programs and measure outcomes.

These caveats notwithstanding, the past twenty years' experimentation with the telephone in health delivery is really quite remarkable. Although we need more research to help us understand the power of the telephone alone and in conjunction with other modalities, the technology is now available to deliver a wide range of health intervention services via the telephone.

The telephone has already shown good results in assessment, monitoring, and providing straightforward interventions to targeted or geographically dispersed populations. There is good evidence that mixing the telephone in with other modalities strengthens the model. The next decade should reveal even better ways to unlock the potential of the telephone in health care delivery, prevention, and management of disease.

References

Anders, G. "Telephone Triage: How Nurses Take Calls and Control the Care of Patients from Afar." *Wall Street Journal*, Feb. 4, 1997.

Balas, F., and others. "Electronic Communication with Patients: Evaluation of Distance Medicine Technology." JAMA: *Journal of the American Medical Association*, July 9, 1997, 278(2), 152–159.

Curry, C., and others. "A Randomized Trial of Self-Help Materials, Personalized Feedback, and Telephone Counseling with Non-volunteer Smokers." *Journal of Consulting Clinical Psychology*, Dec. 1995, 63(6), 1005–1014.

Davis, E., and others. "Evaluation of Three Methods for Improving Mammography Rates in a Managed Care Plan." *American Journal of Preventive Medicine*, July-Aug. 1987, 13(4), 298–302.

Friedman, R. H., and others. "A Telecommunications System for Monitoring and Counseling Patients with Hypertension: Impact on Medication Adherence and Blood Pressure Control." *American Journal of Hypertension*, Apr. 1996, 9(4 Pt 1), 285–292.

Hallam, L. "You've Got a Lot to Answer for, Mr. Bell: A Review of the Use of the Telephone in Primary Care." *Journal of Family Practice*, 1989, 6, 47–57.

King, E., and others. "Promoting Mammography Use Through Progressive Interventions: Is It Effective?" *American Journal of Public Health*, 1994, 84(1), 104–106.

Lynch, Tamburrino, M. B., and Nagel, R. "Telephone Counseling for Patients with Minor Depression: Preliminary Findings in a Family Practice Setting." *Journal of Family Practice*, Mar. 1997, 44(3), 293–298.

Mason, T. "Enhancing Patient Accountability." In W. M. Shaw and D. E. Kolb (eds.), *Managing Integration and Operations: A Guide to Quality Health Care Systems*. New York: Thompson Publishing, 1995.

Mason, T. "Health Promotion Strategies for the Unreachable." *Employee Benefit News,* Apr. 1996, pp. 40–42.

Miller, and others. "Enhancing Adherence Following Abnormal Pap Smears Among Low-Income Minority Women: A Preventive Telephone Counseling Strategy." *Journal of the National Cancer Institute,* May 21, 1989, 10, 703–708.

McConneaughey, J., Nila, C., and Sloan, T. "Falling Through the Net: A Survey of the 'Have Nots' in Rural and Urban America." Department of Commerce, July 1995.

O'Donnell, M. "Health Impact of Workplace Health Promotion." Presentation at Worksite Health 1996 Annual International Conference, Sept. 18–21, 1996, Phoenix, Ariz.

"Patients More Apt to Admit Mental Disorders to Computers Than Physicians." *APA Monitor,* Nov. 1997, pp. 1–2.

"Phone Counseling Services Boom As Health Plans Seek to Curb Costs." *American Medical Association Science News,* Nov. 1995, pp. 5–6.

Rimer, C. T., and others. "Does Tailoring Matter? The Impact of a Tailored Guide on Ratings and Short-Term Smoking Related Outcomes for Older Smokers." *Health Education Research Theory and Practice,* 1994, 1, 69–84.

Siegel, K., and others. "Computerized Telephone Assessment of the 'Concrete' Needs of Chemotherapy Outpatients: A Feasibility Study." *Journal of Clinical Oncology,* Nov. 1988, pp. 1760–1767.

Sleek, S. "Providing Therapy from a Distance." *APA Monitor,* Aug. 1997, pp. 1–4.

Soet, C. B. "The Telephone As a Communication Medium for Health Education." *Health Education and Behavior,* Dec. 1997, 24(6), 759–772.

Wasson, J., and others. "Telephone Care As a Substitute for Routine Clinic Follow-Up." *JAMA: Journal of the American Medical Association,* 1992, 267, 1788–1793.

Zhu, and others. "Telephone Counseling for Smoking Cessation: Effects of a Single Session and Multiple Session Interventions." *Journal of Consulting Clinical Psychology,* Feb. 1996, 64(1), 202–211.

Part III

. . . .

Methods and Options for Behavior
Change Interventions

There are a wide variety of tools and techniques for implementing a health and disease management program. Effective
behavior change interventions may be accomplished by telephone,
as the previous chapter testified, or by any number of nonpersonal
or interpersonal media: publications, audiovisuals, web sites, and
others. More intensive, arguably more effective, and certainly more
costly are the interventions requiring interpersonal contact, such
as individual counseling, case management, classes, and support
groups.

The future may very well belong to health and disease managers
who can find the right balance of high-tech and low-tech tools and
personal and nonpersonal interventions that best serve their
patients' needs and program goals.

Celeste Cafiero and Fern Carness return in Chapter Six to illustrate what it takes to implement successful intervention programs.
First they look at how a national program incorporates elements of
many behavioral change models into a self-controlled systematic
method for quitting smoking. Next, they talk about the importance
of the method chosen to identify potential disease management program participants to avoid alienating those not ready to change.
Assessing participants' readiness to change and health belief systems allows the tailoring of program components to their needs and
interests.

Chapter Seven delves into how information and communication technologies will revolutionize the implementation of health and disease management. Daniel Newton and Neal Sofian expound on a thesis that human relationships will remain the key ingredient to success in the face of rapid technological advancements. Armed with new tools, program architects can move from data to knowledge, from static to dynamic information, and from knowledge to action.

We have only just begun to assemble the comprehensive toolkit with which we will build a brighter future. The methods and options presented in Chapters Six and Seven will have to be continuously tested, refined, and improved for ever more practical and effective use by a new generation of health and disease management programs.

6

Implementing Behavior Change Methods

Celeste Cafiero, Fern Carness

I n Chapter Three we described the various health behavior change models. The observation was made that health care providers responsible for developing successful, measurable disease management efforts ought to consider combining several intervention models to create the "teachable moment" needed for each individual. Here we present strategies that incorporate elements of these models to meet the professed goals of aiding individuals in making and maintaining health behavior change.

Implementing Behavior Change Principles in a Smoking Cessation Program

The American Lung Association's Freedom from Smoking (FFS) program, a nationally developed smoking cessation program, is a well-known program attended by many individuals with chronic diseases. Although it is not a direct component of all disease state management programs, it is a resource to which many patients with diabetes, heart disease, heart failure, chronic obstructive pulmonary disorder, and other conditions are referred as part of their total medical and lifestyle regimen.

The FFS is an eight-session program designed to run over a six-week period. The FFS is resource rich, serving multiple learning styles by providing print, video, and group formats. It is a highly structured group process using a systematic method for quitting smoking and a logical progression from awareness through behavior change as demonstrated by the transtheoretical model. The transtheoretical, or stages of change, model is the predominant model used by the FFS and has influenced the educational design and structure of the program. The FFS focuses on multiple behavior change principles. The methods are positive and directive, not aversive. Many elements of the social learning theory, the theory of planned behavior, and the relapse prevention model can also be identified.

The underlying premise of the FFS is that smoking is a learned habit that becomes an automatic activity. The clinic offers a step-by-step process to change this acquired behavior.

Research shows that 95 percent of all smokers who have successfully quit did so on their own without a formal program—but only when they were ready. The FFS program helps participants establish readiness to change and build toward future self-efficacy by beginning the orientation session with an "Are you ready to quit?" quiz.

Following the principles set forth in the transtheoretical model by Prochaska and DiClemente, the FFS format moves the participant through the stages of change. The program schedule allows adjustment to each stage before moving on to the next, which assists in building self-efficacy and motivation while increasing awareness of the undesirable behavior.

Self-knowledge, observation, and recording are key to successful self-modification. The first session incorporates many self-observation and recording principles used in social learning theory. The use of "Pack Track" forms to record cigarettes smoked uses several behavior change principles. They provide an easy place to record cigarette use because the form fits into the cellophane of the pack and a pencil the same size as a cigarette is provided as well. The form also asks for recording the level of need (addiction) and the mood at the time of the occurrence of the behavior. This information will be helpful in later formulating a plan to control smoking behavior during the cessation process.

Successive approximations, or shaping, can help one to reach the goal of the desired behavior. The second session of the FFS program introduces the concept of nicotine fading—the process of reducing the nicotine level of the cigarettes to decrease addiction gradually. This is a staged approach of small steps over time. Additional shaping features are built into the program: the mere act of rating and recording each cigarette helps bring the action out of the subconscious and into the present, thus shaping the activity of enhanced awareness necessary to combat this behavior. Smoking has several components that need to be addressed at the same time: the physiological, the psychological, and the behavioral. Shaping the behavioral facet occurs when the stimulus is reprogrammed to a new action as in the rating and recording plan.

Many kinds of behavior are learned by observing others. The FFS program encourages the participants to model in several ways. First, they are asked to study nonsmokers and discuss in their groups what nonsmokers do in situations in which smokers tend to pick up a cigarette; for instance, after a meal, in a tense situation, or while waiting. This helps in providing a role model for difficult situations and for practicing or rehearsing what one will do at such times. This element is incorporated into another technique used in the program, that of using a buddy system as a form of support and public declaration. Once again, elements of the self-directed behavior change process including the techniques of stimulus control, social support, and behavior rehearsal are used. In addition, participants are shown videos of smoking rituals and they discuss the observed behavior in small groups. This activity demonstrates the use of the relapse prevention model by having individuals identify and prepare for relapse situations.

Using the group process to learn effective and ineffective quitting techniques helps quitters in devising alternate coping strategies for their successful cessation. Stimulus control is the term given to a set of procedures that seeks to alter the antecedent that controls the unwanted behavior. During the third session, planning for quit day begins with removing all smoking paraphernalia from the home, office, and car. This serves to clean out the physical environment and reduces the most common stimulus or triggers to smoke. In session four the participants complete a "plan ahead" list to identify procedures they will follow when they find themselves in a particular smoking situation. Having multiple options of what they will do instead of smoking will support this new behavior and reinforce the commitment to cessation. This serves as both behavior rehearsal as well as a relapse prevention technique.

Visual cues and positive self-talk can support new behavior. The behavioral component of smoking is triggered by environmental cues, such as talking on the phone, starting the car, or having coffee. The FFS program uses stickers as visual cues to not smoke in the cue environments and teaches several mantras for positive self-talk for these situations, such as: "You're just a puff away from a pack a day" and "The urge to smoke will pass, whether I smoke or not." These are powerful strategies to prevent relapse.

Using a behavioral contract is a behavior change principle that relies on reward and punishment. The FFS program offers a contract—a key self-directed process component—as a tool to reinforce the commitment to stop smoking. This contract is witnessed by the participant's buddy, who provides emotional support for the quitter. The contract has a reward component to serve as a reinforcer that will strengthen the probability that the desired behavior will occur. Using the buddy system here serves to further increase the public nature of the decision to stop smoking.

The FFS promotes a predetermined quit date based on the length of the program. Making this exception to an otherwise self-controlled process is by design, because the literature shows that many smokers will delay setting their quit date or fall prey to the idea that smoking "just a few" is a sustainable new goal. Going back to the stages-of-change model, participants who decide to take action on their desired behavior change by joining the FFS program may still find external quit-date setting intimidating. However, as long as sufficient emphasis is given to trying to quit on that date with contingency plans built in for those who don't make it through the first time, the locus of control remains with the individual and concentrating on success and ultimate maintenance becomes the focus.

In summary, the Freedom from Smoking Program effectively integrates many health behavior change models to offer a variety of approaches and techniques to participants attempting to change their smoking behavior.

Identifying and Stratifying Program Participants

Many health care organizations have launched disease state management programs based on protocols that offer disease-specific programs to those patients identified through pharmacy or claims data. These programs typically incorporate cyclical mailings or phone interventions or both for the purposes of altering health behavior as demonstrated by increased compliance with medication regimen, improved lifestyle habits, or decreased utilization of emergency services or inappropriate physician visits.

What is missing in many of these models is that participants are chosen based only on their utilization patterns or pharmacy data. Such programs frequently do not evaluate participants' readiness to change or their health belief system.

A preferred entrée into a disease management program would be a communication vehicle that assesses the participant's readiness to move from precontemplation to contemplation or from contemplation to preparation, thus advancing along the continuum of change. This technique also provides a needed cue to action that engages the participant early in the change process. In contrast, providing a set menu of resources regardless of the relevance to the participant's personal situation does not create the needed "teachable moment" but, rather, can effectively alienate the participant.

A solid program first identifies potential participants using a quantitative method. The next step is to stratify participants by assessing their readiness to change and evaluating their health belief system. Stratifying a population provides the opportunity to tailor your messages and program components to best suit the current needs and interests of your at-risk population, thereby enhancing the likelihood of moving participants along the behavior change continuum.

Many broad-based disease management programs profess to have behavior change as their goal, yet the key strategies driving program design and implementation are marketing agendas rather than clinical criteria. For example, a predetermined collection of print materials, videos, newsletters, reminder cards, and so on mailed to people identified by prescription data is often ignored because it doesn't meet the recipients' specific needs or interests. In some instances, the superficial design or look of program materials is considered more important than creating an effective educational design that engages the learner. If the criterion for success is patient satisfaction or improved name recognition, then programs with a primary marketing focus can help reach that goal; but they should not be confused with behavior change programs.

Most disease management programs that are preset do offer patients an opportunity to self-select for the program by completing a registration card, calling an 800 number, or returning a survey tool that indicates readiness for the program. These programs enhance a sense of empowerment. Those that automatically enroll a participant based on utilization criteria are running the risk of angering those who are uninterested. If improving compliance or increasing persistency with a medical and lifestyle program is the goal, a more targeted methodology will enhance your opportunity for success. A preferred model would include profiling individual patients for their unique combination of risk, readiness to change, knowledge, and preferred learning styles and providing only those educational elements that are pertinent to them.

Conclusion

With all disease management program planning, remember that creating a systems approach is much more effective than focusing merely on individual-component management. To develop such a system requires fostering self-efficacy in both health care providers and patients. Methods to reach this goal include:

- Educating health care providers on best practices

- Measuring patient interest and readiness to change

- Assisting both patients and health care providers in working and communicating more successfully with each other

- Combining health behavior change models

- Providing tailored messages appropriate to individual participants

- Maintaining a blend of high-tech media and high-touch concepts

- Varying the techniques included to help participants make and sustain behavior change

- Providing incentives for both health care providers and patients

- Increasing the frequency of contact with participants

- Measuring and analyzing data

- Refining the program based on evaluation data

· ·

7

Connecting People and Technologies for Disease Management

Daniel L. Newton, Neal S. Sofian

Like health care itself, disease management in the new millennium will be transformed in ways beyond our ability to predict. Three major forces will be among those at the forefront of this transformation: the changing demographics of our population; amazing advances in technologies associated with medical diagnosis, treatment, and delivery of care; and increased use of combinations of pharmaceutical products, a development that presents new challenges for patient education. This chapter focuses on a fourth major force—the health care consumer's increasing influence as a key driver in the demand for services.

This shift is occurring in part because of the continuing development of new communication and information technologies that provide consumers with the information they need to take a more active role in making decisions about their care. As a result of this shift, the health care industry will become increasingly more concerned with building strong relationships between providers and patients. Stronger bonds can be achieved by applying emerging theories of relationship marketing via those very same communication and information technologies—especially multimedia, which can integrate voice, video, and data. These technologies provide cost-efficient methods for delivering behaviorally based disease management interventions to large numbers of people.

At the same time, health organizations must customize interventions to make them meaningful to individual patients. When organizations do this well, they can form strong and lengthy relationships with large populations of consumers. Such loyal relationships are key to better disease and demand management because they bring about long-term behavior change and patient compliance with care recommendations.

The Evolution of Disease Management

To understand why relationship marketing is so important to disease management, it helps to look at the way the field has evolved. As you can see in Figure 7.1, the first wave was the recognition that through better data technologies, population segments with particular diseases could be identified and enrolled in interventions to lower health costs. The second wave focused on variability in treatment to create better efficiencies and consistency in care by implementing care paths and protocols. In this wave, disease management is heavily reliant on educating and molding physician behavior. In the third wave, the industry began to recognize that patients need a continuum of care. A patient with diabetes, for example, may have problems with depression. If providers expect to improve care outcomes, they must focus on the total care of that individual—not just treatment of diabetes.

We hypothesize that in the next wave of disease management, health systems will begin to view the patient as a customer with whom the provider wants to establish a long-term relationship. With this perspective, there will be a greater emphasis on the needs and desires of patients, as well as a greater focus on communication and other aspects of care that strengthen the patient-provider bond. This approach will incorporate better protocols for what, when, how, and by whom patients are contacted within their overall regimen of care. It is in this realm that marketing and technologies spawned by the marketing industry can become the integrator between patients and their care processes.

Figure 7.1. The Evolution of Disease Management.

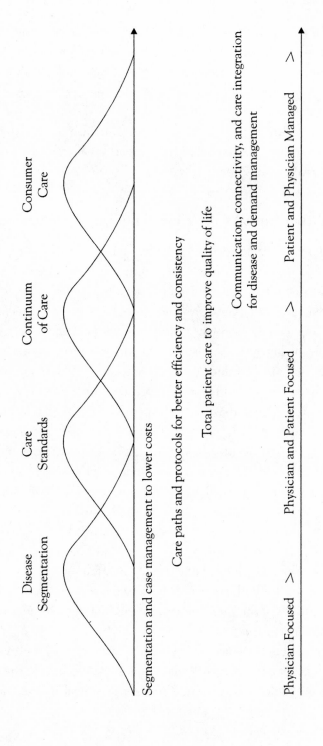

In fact, this focus on communications has been emphasized recently by the Science Panel on Interactive Communication and Health. The panel defined interactive health communications as the interaction of an individual as a consumer, patient, caregiver, or professional with or through an electronic device or communication technology to access or transmit health information or to receive or provide guidance and support on a health-related issue (Science Panel, 1999, p. 8).

Relationships As the Key to Disease Management

In all sectors of business and industry, strategists are focusing on how to build more permanent relationships with customers. Research shows that it costs far more to attract a new customer than to retain an existing one. Therefore companies have become increasingly more focused on customer loyalty (Christopher and others, 1991). While marketers in the past focused primarily on single transactions that emphasized product features, today's brand of relationship marketing emphasizes customer service, commitment, and contact.

Perhaps nowhere is relationship marketing more relevant than in the fields of health care in general and disease management in particular. The health care industry has known for a long time that when patients feel connected to their providers, they are far less likely to switch, regardless of clinical outcomes. Yet it is increasingly more common for patients to switch physicians or even entire modalities of care (from allopathic to naturopathic, for example) if they are not getting the type of support and communication they desire. The financial and practice implications of this trend can be significant for both the providers and payers of care, shaking the foundations of the care delivery systems and the insurance systems that support them.

In her book *Market-Driven Health Care*, Herzlinger (1997) postulates that consumers will place a premium on having the ability to make choice and value trade-offs for their health care. Survivors in the health care industry will be those organizations that create efficient and integrated systems designed to respond to consumer needs. At present, however, she points out that one of the biggest problems with the U.S. health care system is the lack of integration of services, particularly from the customer's perspective. Although many of today's health promotion and wellness efforts are intended to be part of a relationship-building process for health plans and providers, they are usually disconnected from any care process.

At the same time, the line between marketing and care is becoming harder to distinguish. As care becomes more dependent on patient affinity and compliance, its goals seem more congruent with those of marketing. This is an important transition in today's managed care environment where many consumers are dissatisfied with their health care. Because they have less contact with known providers, many feel frightened and alienated from their care system. Some consumers express fear that faceless number crunchers are making decisions about their personal care and, in most cases, recommending less care. This is despite that fact that the U.S. population's health status continues to improve.

Communicating to Inform Patient Choice

How can health systems respond to this sense of alienation? We believe the answer lies in protocols that build affinity, continuity, and integration of care. We must transform the patient-provider relationship by placing greater emphasis on communication, leading consumers to greater choice and involvement in their own care. This more intense relationship can serve two closely related purposes: to improve patients' loyalty to their providers and to influence patients' everyday decisions regarding health behavior like drug compliance and lifestyle issues such as exercise, nutrition, smoking, and stress management—decisions key to disease and demand management.

Stronger patient-provider relationships become possible when health systems interact with patients based on an understanding of how and why people make decisions about their health and health behavior. Providers must pay attention to factors such as individual patients' motivations, barriers, health beliefs, learning style, preferences, and readiness to change.

Given the significance of consumer affinity and choice, we believe that the next wave of advances in disease management will not be the result of new behavioral theories or better technologies, although technology will allow an increase in the number and variety of interventions possible. Rather, the next wave will come through the application of what McKenna (1991) refers to as new marketing models. Such models rely on knowledge-based and experience-based approaches to reaching customers and developing products. Applying these approaches to disease management will mean finding ways to integrate the patient into the care process and creating methods for establishing sustained relationships among consumers, payers, and providers of health care. It also means accepting that all parties—consumers and providers included—play an increasingly significant and collaborative role.

Migration to New Communication Technologies

As disease management and marketing become more closely aligned, health programs will benefit by adopting many of the same communication technologies that are transforming the field of marketing. Advances in computer hardware and software have increased our ability to integrate, manage, and manipulate enormous amounts of information. By some estimates, the speed of computing doubles every twelve to eighteen months at the same time the cost of hardware declines by half (Van Brunt, 1998). Advances in the development of sophisticated rule-based programming—also called expert systems—now allow us to instantly and automatically find, tailor, and deliver very specific pieces of information to individual providers and patients that can make a critical difference in patient care. And in the very near future, an even more sophisticated level of programming will be available to health care, one that goes beyond the rule-based systems to heuristic systems. Also referred to as artificial intelligence, these systems automatically change and grow in response to the data patterns that emerge as databases of consumer transactions grow in size.

In marketing, such information technology is being used increasingly to segment groups of potential buyers according to their readiness to purchase and other psychodemographic characteristics. Marketers can then determine the best timing and frequency of their sales contacts based on these profiles. Similar strategies are being applied to health behavior change, allowing program developers to design better protocols for disease management. Much like a sales contact-management tool, such protocols can determine the most appropriate timing and frequency for communicating with particular segments of the population. Based on psychodemographic assessments of patients, we can design protocols for particular segments of our population, using the communication channel, tailored message, and delivery style that is most appropriate for those groups. For instance, a contact protocol may tell us when to send a letter versus a phone call or may determine that a patient prefers e-mail to conventional mail. Taking it one step further, tailored messages can actually be constructed based on whether a patient responds better to stories or simple fact sheets.

Increased consumer access to computers via the Internet and interactive voice response (IVR) telephone systems is hastening our ability to apply these marketing strategies. According to the *eMarketer* overview report, approximately 28.7 percent of all U.S. adults over the age of eighteen (approximately 58 million Internet users) were actively using the Internet by the end of 1999. Such usage is expected to grow to 42.2 percent by 2002. One of the fastest growing segments of Internet users are teens, which will grow at an annualized rate of 63 percent between 1999 and 2002 compared with the adult usage growth rate of 23 percent. Such growth will produce unprecedented means for demand and disease managers to reach these populations with messages and programs for prevention and health improvement ("eOverview Report," 2000, pp. 16–20).

Research also shows that increasing numbers of people are using the Internet for health-related purposes. Some 52 percent of people with on-line access searched for health information in 1997. In March 1998, there were an estimated 250,000 health-related web sites, not including Usenet newsgroups devoted to health issues (Junnarkar, 1998). In addition, a large percentage of health plan members now have access to the Internet. In 1998 it was estimated that approximately 45 percent of all U.S. households had computers (Science Panel, 1999, p. 7) and in 1999 there were 29.7 million households that had on-line connections to the Internet ("eOverview Report," 2000, p. 45).

With such widespread consumer access to systems that converge database information and communication technologies, the health care industry has the opportunity to increase the reach and richness of their disease management programs as never before. Such technologies can be used to create "physician extenders," expanding a single provider's ability to efficiently reach larger numbers of patients. One simple example is the physician who communicates with his or her patients via e-mail. As use of Internet technology evolves, patients and providers may begin to use real audio or video clips, thus adding back some of the value lost by not having in-person health care visits.

Health care systems' migration to new communication technologies alters the challenges for disease management in many ways. Rather than focusing on the problem of patients' access to health information, for example, today's health care providers would do well to focus on the manner and style in which information is delivered. As we thus adapt technology to account for how people learn and act on what they learn, the art of communication will play a more significant role in disease management.

Technology Adoption and Change

Although new communication technologies hold great promise for disease management in the new millennium, our success at effectively integrating them into the health care system will depend greatly on our ability to help consumers and providers adapt to change. Often there is a huge gap between what is technologically possible and what is pragmatically implemented. Every new technology comes with a behavioral boundary that often limits its adoption and assimilation into the mainstream. Just because technology provides common-sense solutions doesn't mean all people are willing to use them. Barriers are particularly strong when use requires people to change their habits. Think Beta versus VHS, or Apple Computer versus the PC. And in health care, think paper versus electronic medical records (EMRs).

Electronic Medical Records

Technologically, EMRs can streamline records and create an integrated patient medical information system. But getting physicians and others to change how they record, access, and use medical records in order to make this possible has turned out to be a tremendous hurdle.

Overcoming such behavioral boundaries is addressed in Moore's book *Crossing the Chasm: Marketing and Selling High-Tech Products to Mainstream Customers* (1991). Describing waves in the product adoption cycle, Moore points to a huge chasm between the way what he terms early adopters and the early majority successfully adapt to new technology. While the early adopters like to take risks, the early majority look for proven ways to improve what they are currently doing. Engaging the early majority requires completely different strategies from engaging the early adopters. As Moore explains, innovation and the next wave of change occur when technology makes it easier for consumers to perform a behavior they are used to doing.

The Internet

Amazon.com, the on-line bookseller, is one example of a company that provides a convenient new way for consumers to do something they've always done—in this case, buying books. Amazon understands that consumers have become increasingly comfortable with catalog purchases of consumer goods. Based on the idea that the best change is none (or as little as possible), Amazon eliminated the paper catalog but left the process of browsing (albeit on the Internet) intact. Now that the company has established a relationship with consumers as a seller of books, music CDs, and videos, Amazon is introducing other, less tangible products and services.

Searching for health information is another common activity made easier through the technology of the Internet. Logging on to a health information site such as The Mayo Clinic's Mayo Health-O@sis (www.mayohealth.org) or Johns Hopkins' InteliHealth (www.intelihealth.com) is far more convenient than traveling to the library and searching through shelves of books.

Automatic Teller Machines

Often we become comfortable with the most sophisticated technology by using it to access low-tech products and services with which people are already familiar. One example is paper currency. We have been using it for hundreds of years and are not yet ready to abandon it for a totally plastic debit-credit system. Still, we're using automatic teller machines (ATMs) with increasing frequency as a preferred way to acquire cash and monitor our account balances. It is a marvel to many (and a terror to some) to know that a $50 ATM withdrawal not only provides you with cash, but immediately updates all of your accounts as well. The ATM system ensures that you only take a certain amount and it monitors your transactions to detect illegal use of your card. Without the communication technology to back up the ATM, we might still be going to the bank to deposit or cash our checks.

Telephonic Interactive Voice Response

We are also comfortable with the telephone. And now, with telephonic IVR programs, people are using their phone keypads and voices to send and receive information directly to computer networks. Physicians at Allina Health Systems' rural Minnesota facilities, for example, no longer have emergency room duty because of the health systems' investment in telemedicine technologies. Board-certified emergency physicians at a Buffalo, Minnesota, facility now perform video consults with Allina patients throughout the region. HealthPartners, a Minneapolis-based HMO, is using videophones to replace home-care visits. Using the videophone, nurses can view measurements of a patient's heart rate, blood pressure, and other biometric data as well as see how a wound is healing (Tweed, 1998).

Value Creation in Disease Management

What lessons do such examples provide for disease management in the new millennium? We must draw our cues from existing care delivery systems and the ways in which patients and providers traditionally interact. For example, patients who go to their personal care providers for help with diabetes management expect to get more than one-size-fits-all advice. Consciously or unconsciously, providers broadly assess the individual patient's situation and tailor the interaction based on a variety of factors. If the provider does a good job, patients will become more knowledgeable about the disease and be inspired to take action on their own behalf, perhaps improving diet, exercise, and glucose monitoring habits.

Using technology to improve and leverage these highly personalized interactions—effectively extending provider reach and influencing consumer behavior—will require key transitions in disease management. Specifically, new technology must use data to impart knowledge as opposed to mere information; information must become dynamic, personalized, and interactive as opposed to the static forms currently available on many health-related web sites;

and new knowledge must motivate people toward health action and health-related transactions. If we do these things, we can ensure that the changes technology requires represent a solid value proposition. In other words, we can prove that the advantages of using computers, IVR, and other tools outweigh their disadvantages, whatever those might be.

This trade-off certainly comes into play when we ask consumers to share personal health data—a request that often raises concerns about privacy and use of data. Confidential health information is often key to personalizing computer-based interventions and making them more effective. How do health systems address such concerns? We believe the privacy issue reflects whether consumers value what they get in return for the information they are asked to share. A personally tailored health intervention that can help a person make a desired but difficult change in health behavior might be worth the perceived risk of sharing confidential data. Unless consumers perceive such value, however, problems can ensue. We see evidence of this with supermarket club cards that are being distributed as a way to track customers' purchases and offer targeted promotions. Some consumers, who apparently feel that receiving the promotions is not worth the loss of privacy regarding their purchases, have chosen to boycott retailers issuing the cards.

The relative value of sharing health information electronically may also need to be addressed by lawmakers as they consider restricting Internet use, telemedicine applications, and other electronic means of channeling medical information. Unless the value to society is clear, legal restrictions may continue as barriers to consumer use of new technology for disease management.

Ultimately, new communication technologies will become highly valued tools for disease management for at least three reasons: they will help disease management programs move from dealing in data to dealing in knowledge; they will allow us to deliver dynamic, rich, personalized information instead of static information; and they will allow us to turn knowledge into action.

Moving from Data to Knowledge

Health systems have always collected information about their trans-actions with consumers through medical records, pharmacy claims, and more. Stored and analyzed alone, such discrete databases are no more than electronic filing cabinets; they can't tell organizations that much about the people in their populations and their utiliza-tion, risks, and needs. But now, because of recent advances in data integration and statistical tools, health care systems can combine data from many sources, including medical claims, pharmacy claims, health risk appraisals, personal medical records, and even employee absenteeism and health programming records. This allows organi-zations to create individual and population profiles, enabling them to gain important insights about utilization rates and costs of car-ing for groups of consumers as well as the individual people in those groups. These organizations can then stratify their populations based on expected outcomes and costs, using the knowledge gained from such analysis for resource optimization.

Edington, dean of the University of Michigan's Health Man-agement Research Center, and Tze-ching Yen have done landmark work in this area, developing highly refined stratification models that use algorithms to identify potential high utilizers based on lifestyle-related data (Edington and Tze-ching Yen, 1997). Such tools make it possible for a payer to assign health care–cost trends to each person in its population and then design intervention strate-gies based on future needs and expenses. These systems help health plans, employers, and others monitor, plan, and implement disease management and health promotion interventions.

Today's advanced database technology also allows organizations to analyze health care costs and utilization through comparisons with external databases. Through health care information firms, organizations can have access to databases representing health care services for millions of people. Such broad-based information is use-ful as organizations monitor outcomes and form strategies for man-aging and predicting the utilization and cost of various treatments.

Although these data systems may seem advanced for health care, a look at other industry achievements—particularly in the realm of consumer marketing—gives a hint of things to come. The supermarket club cards mentioned earlier that track purchases are one example and credit card companies are another. With sophisticated data management tools to profile consumers' use patterns and buying behavior, credit card companies can combat fraud by alerting their customers when abnormal use patterns are recognized.

Development of the ability to track transactional patterns in case management and other health care areas is still in its infancy. But we are already seeing how advanced pattern recognition and data management can help the pharmaceutical industry track prescription drug usage. Companies are now networking pharmacies and acting as agents to actively follow up with consumers who haven't picked up their medications or who should be renewing their prescriptions. Imagine if health plans had this level of sophistication and could use health assessment data to flag future problems related to changing patterns in your diet, weight, use of medicine, or physician visits. Health systems could be alerted to intervene with patients or groups of patients before problems got out of hand. A lot of energy and research dollars are being spent on systems like Edington's Trend Management System for this exact purpose.

Advances in the development of computerized health risk appraisals (HRAs) now provide health systems with efficient ways to collect and integrate risk information. With the right programming, such information can be instantly matched to tailored messages that are designed to help the consumer reduce risks.

Consumers typically have access to computerized HRAs via the Internet or telephone using an IVR touch-tone system. Either method allows data to be transmitted directly and instantly into an organization's computer. And in the future, health systems may use satellite transmissions for the same purpose. A patient could complete an HRA in the provider's office, using the type of hand-held device that United Parcel Service drivers use to keep track of packages. His or her health system's computers could then receive satellite transmissions of the data and report it to a large database where it would be analyzed to predict future risk. The computer could then generate a report, which would instantly be transmitted back to the clinic, for the patient to discuss with the provider.

Such systems often store information from HRAs so that later they can initiate reminders about health screenings and future appointments. Systems might even be programmed to send e-mail and voice mail to the patient to encourage compliance.

Although the 1990s have been dubbed "the decade of information overload," disease management has benefited from the explosion in information technology. It has allowed consumers to become active players in their care and it has provided the health care industry with a basis for better patient targeting and management. Transforming information to knowledge in the new millennium will require that we become smarter about determining what information is really useful for decision making and program development. This will call for more foresight as well as a more analytical approach to data. With all this data at our fingertips, we must keep in mind that more is not necessarily better. Gathering and processing information require time, and time is a valued resource of both consumers and providers. Drucker (1998, p. 68) writes, "Knowledge constantly makes itself obsolete, with the result that today's advanced knowledge is tomorrow's ignorance." Keeping up with the shelf-life of knowledge when information access is constantly expanding will place new pressures on all parties involved in the care process.

Moving from Static to Dynamic Information

As patients and providers become more knowledgeable about disease and care processes, disease management programs using technology will focus more on delivery processes than on content. Programs in the midst of this transition need to pay increasing attention to the concepts of richness and reach. Evans and Wurster (1997) discuss these concepts in a *Harvard Business Review* article entitled "Strategy and the Economics of Information":

> To the extent that information is embedded in physical modes of delivery, its economics are governed by a basic law: the trade-off between richness and reach. Reach simply means the number of the people, at home or at work, exchanging information. Richness is defined by three aspects of the information itself. The first is bandwidth, or the amount of information that can be moved from sender to receiver in a given time. Stock quotes are narrowband; a film is broadband. The second aspect is the degree to which the information is customized. For example, an advertisement on television is far less personally customized than a personal sales pitch but reaches far more people. The third aspect is interactivity. Dialogue is possible for a small group, but to reach millions of people the message must be a monologue [p. 73].

Because so much of disease management is rooted in behavior change, it depends greatly on the nonclinical tools of information exchange and communication. Tools such as telephone call centers, interactive voice response systems, newsletters, the Internet, and CD ROMs can all be useful. And through advances in information technology, all of these tools are being transformed in ways that can expand the reach and richness of the information they deliver.

Telephone Call Centers

Telephone call centers are not new to health care. Nurses have been taking inbound calls for the purpose of demand management at various centers for more than twenty years. In fact, most large health plans now provide phone-based advice to consumers (Connolly, 1996) because studies show such calls can reduce demand for outpatient services (Lazarus, 1995). A new trend has emerged, however, with call centers providing outbound calls aimed at disease management and behavior change. The power of using outbound call centers for behavior change was proven in 1986 in a National Cancer Institute study of Group Health Cooperative of Puget Sound's Free & Clear smoking intervention, which achieved twelve-month quit rates as high as 34 percent (Orleans and others, 1991). Depending on the type of help needed, call center services may be delivered by a range of professionals, such as nurses, counselors, or behavior change facilitators. Participants receive calls at home or work, getting help with drug regimens, chronic medical conditions such as diabetes and asthma, or difficult behavior changes such as smoking cessation and weight control.

Currently, most telephone-based intervention programs are quite similar to traditional classroom-based behavior change programs. Programs of the future, however, will become increasingly more powerful through the use of assessments to determine a wide range of psychodemographic characteristics. Assessments can be used to identify specific learning and behavior styles as well as hobbies and effective metaphors for learning. Powered by such data, telephonic and other remote technologies may demonstrate potent outcomes, perhaps even stronger than face-to-face interventions.

In the nonmedical world, call centers have become big business and are key components of sales, marketing, brand management, and customer service strategies. Because of their widespread customer reach, call centers have become an essential part of any strategy involving customer relationships. As in many other areas of health care, we believe that disease management is just catching up with more consumer-focused industries and benefiting from the lessons therein.

In the same way, health systems are just now recognizing and acting on the strategic link between their call center activities, physician and patient relationships, and overall approach to population care processes. For example, systems have only recently begun to integrate their nurse call lines with their disease management and appointment scheduling capabilities. Still, the importance and proliferation of call centers in health care is growing.

Tailored Health Communication

Just as telephone call centers can deliver rich, personalized interventions to large segments of a population, so too can various forms of tailored communication, now available in a variety of media, including print, IVR phone systems, and the Internet. Tailored health communication is an enhancement of disease management initially made possible through advances in mail-merge functionality and proliferated through developments in database and printing technology. Tailoring takes population targeting and segmentation—by-products of health risk appraisals—even further to create "segments of one"; that is, designing interventions to fit each individual's unique set of characteristics and needs.

Tailored interventions have been proven effective in several investigations, including those involving smoking cessation (Strecher and others, 1994), breast cancer screening (Skinner, Strecher, and Hospers, 1994, pp. 43–49), and dietary change and exercise (Brug and others, 1996). Most studies of tailoring to date have involved tailored print newsletters, but a few organizations are also developing interventions for other media, such as the Internet and telephonic IVR. Examples include WellMed (1998), a company based in Portland, Oregon, that uses an on-line HRA to provide users with customized web links, pointing them to personally relevant health information sites. RealAge (1998), another Internet provider of HRAs, is using the HRA to push relevant health messages to users via e-mail.

While the web can deliver tailored information in an efficient way, IVR provides an especially promising channel for tailored messaging because of the population's widespread access to touch-tone telephones. In addition to simply collecting information via an IVR-based HRA, such systems can be programmed to facilitate ongoing automated interactions between patients and providers. For example, systems can be set to contact patients regarding medication regimens, their own behavior change goals, or upcoming screening exams. Providers also can use IVR to answer consumers' questions with a series of the providers' own prerecorded responses. Using tailoring software, providers can mix and match those responses, creating speeches personally designed for a specific need at a specific time.

In addition, providers may point their patients to an audio library of longer, prerecorded programs covering a range of health-related topics. Audio libraries are beginning to experiment with a variety of innovative formats. For example, HealthTalk Interactive (1998), a Seattle-based company, creates a variety of interactive telephone and Internet "talk shows" featuring experts and lay-people discussing topics such as asthma, headaches, multiple sclerosis, prostate cancer, and kidney disease. Shows are produced in a familiar call-in radio talk show format, allowing people to share resources, information, and, most important, stories of how they have lived with health problems or made changes in health behavior. Tapes of the show are then edited and stored by topic for other individuals to access by phone or computer. The format supports personalized and intimate communication that can inspire life changes. At the same time, it extends the reach of those discussions, as previously recorded conversations become available to thousands.

With tailored messaging, organizations are acknowledging that often effectiveness in communication is more related to how a message is delivered and received by the listener than to the content of the message. In other words, part of making health behavior change interventions more appealing is to better match patients to programs, looking not only at how they like to receive information, but also at how they are most likely to be "moved" by information. The authors of this chapter are principals of The NewSof Group, a Seattle-based consulting firm that is helping organizations use new technologies to develop more effective behavior change interventions. We like to categorize how people typically approach behavior change in three different ways: planning, tracking, and storytelling. This planner, tracker, storyteller model is built on the understanding that there is no shortage of information in most fields of health behavior change. There is, however, a lack of insight about how to motivate people to take action.

Planners change by looking forward, setting goals, making plans, and following those plans until they achieve their goals. Trackers change by keeping records of their behavior and then looking back and analyzing patterns. They then adjust their behavior based on what they learn from that retrospective reflection. Storytellers neither plan nor track. Instead, they find the inspiration and strength to change after sharing anecdotes and testimonials with others. Oprah Winfrey–style, they are first attracted by the emotional appeal of a personal story and then follow up by gathering information and strategies to make change.

We believe that classic behavior modification techniques—which include goal setting, tracking, and rewards for progress—can work well for the planners and trackers. But storytellers may benefit from new and different forms of intervention that allow participants to share their own stories and listen to the stories of others. Patients can be encouraged to share their experiences on Internet bulletin boards, in their own journals, or by taking photos to create a picture story of their barriers to making change. Phone counselors can urge storytellers to see movies, watch television programs, or listen to tapes with narratives related to themes of behavior change. High-quality entertainment can arouse emotions, causing people to see their behavior in new ways. Storytellers may also be able to participate in interactive health "talk shows," described earlier and made available via telephone IVR systems and Internet "real audio." They can be encouraged to read about people just like themselves in tailored newsletters and web pages. In this way, they are able to harness the emotional power that music, video, and personally relevant storytelling have to inspire and transform.

All of this speaks to ensuring that patients have the opportunity whenever possible to learn in their own preferred style and medium. Ideally, tailored interventions of the future will be offered in a variety of integrated modalities. That is the intent of the American Heart Association (AHA) as it works with North Carolina–based Micromass, Inc., to deliver "Change of Heart," a tailored intervention aimed at making lifestyle changes to reduce the risk of heart disease (interview by the authors with David Bulger at Micromass, April 1998). After participants in this program complete a health-risk and lifestyle assessment over the phone or Internet, the AHA sends them a printed kit that is tailored by stage of change and a highly tailored print- or web-based quarterly newsletter. The program also includes phone calls and reminder postcards or e-mail messages based on the participants' stage of change during their most recent phone-based counseling session.

Interactive Support

While tailoring helps to make communication more personalized and rich for users, so too does the addition of interactivity. It makes sense, then, that many organizations are using new technologies to create on-line and IVR-based support groups that promote dialogue among consumers with similar health interests.

Research continues to prove the importance of social support in changing behavior and managing disease. Studies conclude, for example, that social support helps people in health crises feel a better sense of control in their lives (Krause, 1987), helping them cope with or adjust to health problems (Taylor and others, 1984). Strong social support can also reduce patients' feelings of anxiety or hopelessness (DiPasquale, 1990). Now, with the advent of outbound telephone call centers, interactive voice response systems, and computerized bulletin boards, consumers have easy access to the kind of social support that was once available only through group meetings and one-to-one counseling.

People who share the same chronic medical conditions or who face similar challenges of making difficult behavior change can now find one another through thousands of on-line bulletin boards and chat rooms devoted to various specific health topics.

IVR-based support systems are gaining in popularity as well. Consisting of a voice mailbox that is shared by a specific group, these IVR systems are usually simple to use. A member of a smoking cessation group, for example, might call the system with a question about symptoms of nicotine withdrawal. The member might be invited to record the question in an area devoted to that topic. Then, when the next member calls and chooses a similar topic, he may hear the first caller's question and respond to it. This action then signals the system to alert the first caller that someone has responded to her question. The system might also tell the caller about other messages recently added to the mailbox. All communication on such systems is confidential; callers are not given one another's names or phone numbers.

IVR support systems can be a real boon to consumers who don't have a computer and can't attend support group meetings. In fact, in a Cleveland State University study of drug-abusing pregnant women, participants were eight time more likely to use the phone-based system than attend face-to-face support group meetings (Alemi and others, 1996). The group who participated in the IVR program also had lower outpatient utilization rates, without bad effects related to health status or drug use.

Such studies point to the advantages that technology-based sources of support can provide over traditional forms. IVR and on-line groups are not limited by participants' schedules or locations. Also, participants can be anonymous, which enables many to feel more comfortable sharing sensitive details of their lives with group members.

Integrated Support Programs

The reach of the support group concept can be extended even further through the use of "virtual support groups," a concept being explored jointly by The NewSof Group and the American Cancer

Society (ACS). In this case, participants can use a toll-free number twenty-four hours a day to access the Cancer Survivors' Network. This IVR- and Internet-based program includes fourteen topical discussions categorized for long-term survivors, newly diagnosed cancer survivors, and caregivers. Listeners hear real cancer survivors telling their stories and providing supportive advice. Callers also can be connected to ACS's National Cancer Information Center for further information and support. In the ACS system, the overriding mantra is that all information for cancer survivors will come from other cancer survivors. All experts used in the recorded sessions are themselves cancer survivors.

Participants can access the ACS program by a touch-tone telephone or the Internet through the use of a computer audio card. The same content is provided in both channels. With the Internet, however, participants can be hot-linked to experts who have participated in the service as well as other organizations delivering care and support. In addition, when users choose the Internet version of the program, the overall cost of delivering the program is lower.

It is possible for IVR systems like the one described above to be integrated with other services. That is because the system not only tracks usage, but also creates a detailed accounting of which segments users found interesting. This IVR data could be used to generate tailored print materials with customization based on which segments each individual chose to hear. To create further support with little cost, tailored letters could be sent to participants informing them of other participants who have similar problems and/or interests and want to be part of a support group. Such groups could manifest themselves as computer- or telephone-based chat groups or as in-person support groups. All would be self-generating and regulated by the participants at no cost to the delivery system.

The ACS program is committed to the concept of personal storytelling as a means of communicating and changing behavior. In the area of chronic disease management, information is essential but insufficient to meet patient needs. Nor can the network rely on information alone to reach the health care delivery system's desired outcomes. We believe it is no accident that more people watch and listen to Oprah than educational TV. In order to achieve the richness of communication that is required for meaningful change, we must learn to appeal to the gut as well as the brain.

In addition to increasing the reach and richness of communication through tailored print, IVR, and the Internet, interventions produced as CD ROMs and video games also deserve notice—especially because of their appeal to the learning preferences of teens and children. Click Health, Inc., of Mountain View, California, is developing a series of video games in Super Nintendo format to help teach children to better self-manage their health, particularly in disease states like asthma. This form of patient education is clearly focusing on the needs of the market segment (children) and the way this segment likes to receive information (computer games and television). The mission of a game for asthma patients is to keep dinosaur characters called "Bronkie" and "Trakie" from coughing and wheezing, while combating an environment filled with smoke, dust, and pollen. This multimedia intervention is being studied to see if it ultimately can reduce asthma attacks in children (Chase, 1998).

Moving from Knowledge to Action

It is great to describe cutting-edge technology that can integrate disease management techniques into seamless delivery systems with a mind-boggling capacity to mine data and provide tailored, high-impact interventions. But with much of this technology still under development, how can we tell what really works? And even more important, what type of map or model can we presently use to help us know if we are moving in the right direction?

Doug Goldstein, a nationally recognized health care consultant (in discussion with the authors, October 1998), is concerned about Internet technologies and how we need to better integrate information with transactional opportunities. When consumers visit a health plan's web site to review the professional backgrounds of its physicians, for instance, wouldn't it be nice if they could make an appointment with the chosen physician during that same inquiry process? When communication technologies are able to satisfactorily meet the customer's full set of needs during each health-related transaction, we'll know these systems are on the right track.

To achieve this level of service, health systems must operate from a truly consumer-oriented perspective, using communication technology to link information, medical access, and transactions within the capabilities of a single channel. Before users finish their connections, they will have been able to get everything they need to take the most appropriate action for themselves.

As an example, let's imagine that I recently learned that my son has diabetes. After using the web to search information sources to learn about diabetes, I might want to view choices for local endocrinologists and schedule an appointment. I might also want to purchase books on diabetes and a glucose-monitoring device. In addition, I may want to link to a family support and parent education site that notifies a diabetes educator to contact me and initiate an education and support process. From a behavioral perspective, each of these steps is viewed as a behavior or an outcome. From a marketing perspective, however, these actions are viewed as transactions. That is, being able to book an appointment, enter into education and support, and make a purchase all in one place are examples of meeting a broader set of consumer needs more efficiently. When technology is created and deployed for its own sake—and primarily focused on the information gathering for early technology adopters—it rarely gets us to these transactional moments of truth. Therefore, in using new technologies to serve consumer needs, we must always ask ourselves two questions:

- Is the technology creating a barrier or facilitating a desired consumer behavior?

- Are we using technology to integrate and meet multiple consumer needs that facilitate a consumer transaction?

On the surface, these points may seem to have little to do with health care. Yet they are the key to how we change our thinking, which in turn will allow us to create systems that can truly support our health care customers to take positive action on their own behalf.

To be most effective, health systems must begin to combine the functions of tailoring, call centers, and the Internet delivery channels, spawning new approaches to health communication and disease management efforts. Imagine a consumer searching a health system web site for information about a disease. She hits a button that links her to a live-call operator who can provide immediate information or behavioral counseling. During that call, the operator gathers additional data and generates a tailored information piece, which is immediately e-mailed to her and her physician. That same information goes into her medical record, so that her provider notes it during a routine visit and uses it to guide communication during the visit. In this scenario interactivity begins to take shape as a result of the initial rich exchange of the information.

Although many health care organizations across the United States are experimenting with different ways to integrate technology to meet consumer needs, one stands out as a particularly good example. That is Celebration Health, an Orlando-based Disney subsidiary that operates a multispecialty health center in Celebration, Florida—Disney's planned "community of tomorrow" (Cross, 1997).

Because their health system's specialty center databases are so well integrated, residents of Celebration can use the Internet on their own home computers to complete a wide variety of health-related transactions. For example, they can book health care appointments, send messages to their doctors, view hospital bills, request information from an electronic health library, and even see most of their own health records. They can also use the health system's database to complete an HRA, which results in periodic personalized e-mail messages. Residents with hay fever, for example, might get news about pollen counts during allergy season. In the future, Celebration Health hopes to provide video links to homes so providers can do virtual house calls, assessing patients' injuries or illnesses while the patients stay comfortably at home.

Conclusion

Celebration Health's rich, integrated, dynamic communication system gives us a glimmer of what is possible when we approach disease management intending to build systems that support long-term relationships with patients. It is a stance that has become increasingly common in nearly every sector of business and industry, heightening expectations among health care consumers as well.

To be successful in the new millennium, disease management programs must learn to apply emerging theories of relationship marketing. When we view healthy behavior change as the product, patients as the customers, and health care providers as the sales force, it is clear that closing the sale requires a strong relationship between buyer and seller. To capitalize on this transformation, we must:

- Focus on the reach and richness of information

- Think of behavior as a transaction

- Find ways to facilitate transactions so that we "close the sale" with a health action or medical event

- Focus on what people do, not what they say

- Start with the person, not the risk

Technology will be at the forefront of interactions between the patient and the provider. Facilitating consumer-oriented transactions for the purpose of creating sustainable relationships related to medical self-care and disease management is the next wave in our approach to more integrated and consumer-focused care.

References

Alemi, F., and others. "Electronic Self-Help and Support Groups." *Medical Care*, 1996, 34(suppl 10).

Brug, J., and others. "The Impact of a Computer Tailored Nutrition Intervention." *Preventive Medicine*, 1996, 25, 236–242.

Chase, M. "Can Video Dinosaurs Help Children Manage Illnesses Like Asthma?" *Wall Street Journal*, Oct. 5, 1998, p. B1.

Christopher, M., and others. *Relationship Marketing: Bringing Quality, Customer Service and Marketing Together*. Oxford: Butterworth, Heinemann, 1991.

Connolly, J. "More Managed Care Plans Add Nurse Phone Lines." *National Underwriter*, Apr. 29, 1996.

Cross, M. A. "Disney's City of the Future." *Health Data Management*, Oct. 1997.

DiPasquale, J. A. "The Psychological Effects of Support Groups on Individuals Infected by the AIDS Virus." *Cancer Nursing*, 1990, 13(5), 278–285.

Drucker, P. *Peter Drucker on the Profession of Management*. Boston: Harvard Business School Press, 1998.

Edington, D., and Tze-ching Yen, L. "The Financial Impact of Changes in Personal Health Practices." *Journal of Environmental Medicine*, Nov. 1997, 39(11), 1037–1046.

"The eOverview Report: Transforming Information into Intelligence." *EMarketer*, Feb. 2000, 2.

Evans, P. B., and Wurster, T. S. "Strategy and the Economics of Information." *Harvard Business Review*, Sept.-Oct., 1997.

HealthTalk Interactive web site (www.htinet.com). Apr. 1998.

Herzlinger, R. *Market-Driven Health Care: Who Wins, Who Loses in the Transformation of America's Largest Service Industry*. Reading, Mass.: Addison-Wesley, 1997.

Junnarkar, S. "Web Sites Warn: Healthcare Information May Not Be What the Doctor Ordered." *New York Times*, Mar. 8, 1998.

Krause, N. "Understanding the Stress Process: Linking Social Support with Locus of Control Beliefs." *Journal of Gerontology*, 1987, 42(6), 589–593.

Lazarus, I. "Medical Call Centers: An Effective Demand Management Strategy for Providers and Plans." *Managed Healthcare*, Oct. 1995, 5(10), 56–59.

McKenna, R. "Marketing Is Everything." *Harvard Business Review*, Jan.-Feb. 1991, pp. 3–10.

Moore, G. A. *Crossing the Chasm: Marketing and Selling High-Tech Products to Mainstream Customers*. New York: HarperCollins, 1991.

Orleans, C. T., and others. "Self-Help Quit Smoking Interventions: Effects of Self-Help Materials, Social Support Instructions, and Telephone

Counseling." *Journal of Consulting and Clinical Psychology*, 1991, 59(3), 439–448.

RealAge corporate web site (www.RealAge.com). Sept. 1998.

Science Panel on Interactive Communication and Health, U.S. Department of Health and Human Services. T. R. Eng and D. H. Gustafson (eds.), *Wired for Health and Well-Being: The Emergence of Interactive Health Communications*. Washington, D.C.: U.S. Government Printing Office, 1999.

Skinner, C. S., Strecher, V. J., and Hospers, H. "Physicians' Recommendations for Mammography: Do Tailored Messages Make a Difference?" *American Journal of Public Health*, Jan. 1994, 84(1).

Strecher, V. J., and others. "The Effects of Computer-Tailored Smoking Cessation Messages in Family Practice Settings." *Journal of Family Practice*, Sept. 1994, 39(3).

Taylor, S. E., and others. "Attributions, Beliefs About Control, and Adjustment to Breast Cancer." *Journal of Personality and Social Psychology*, 1984, 46(3), 489–502.

Tweed, V. "The Brave New World of Telemedicine." *Business & Health*, Sept. 1998.

Van Brunt, D. "Internet-Based Patient Information Systems: What Are They, Why Are They Here, How Will They Be Used, and Will They Work?" *Managed Care Quarterly*, 1998, 6(1), 16–22.

WellMed corporate web site (www.WellMed.com). Sept. 1998.

Part IV

$\bullet \quad \bullet$

Process and Outcome Measurement and Interpretation

The subtitle of this book is *Improving Outcomes in Health and Disease Management*, and so this final section at last affords an in-depth look at how to measure the results of behavior change interventions, both outside and within the context of health or disease management systems. Equally important is understanding how to interpret the results and apply this knowledge to improve the disease management system.

Today, there is little agreement as to what a disease management program should measure to most accurately gauge the outcomes of its efforts. Advances in outcome measurement and interpretation will fuel this ongoing debate and help focus new development efforts in the years ahead.

Chapter Eight presents a primer in basic measurement techniques, results interpretation, and continuous program enhancement. Michael Toscani and Laura Pizzi review the methods for evaluating the effectiveness of the behavior change initiative, interpreting the results of such an evaluation, and applying those interpretations in modifying both the behavior management intervention and the disease management intervention as a whole. The authors answer several questions: Why measure disease management interventions? What should be measured? When should the outcomes of the intervention be measured? They illustrate their measurement and improvement process with a case study involving diabetes disease management interventions.

Careful to distinguish process data from outcome data, Joseph Biskupiak in Chapter Nine expounds on the points raised by Toscani and Pizzi by helping us select the key variables and constructs we need to measure outcomes and shows how these concepts are today being put into practice in successful programs for conditions as diverse as obesity, hypertension, diabetes, and asthma.

Reading these chapters does not complete but, rather, recommences our journey toward improved outcomes in health and disease management. We are prepared to revisit the foundational theories and models with new insights gained from experience. We are again prepared to proceed step by step from theory to practice via proven interventions for changing health-related behavior. And we must be prepared to begin the whole journey yet again in a spirit of continuous improvement.

. . . .

8

Measuring and Improving
the Intervention

Michael R. Toscani, Laura T. Pizzi

Measurement is a key component of any health and disease management system. Without the ability to measure the changes in process and outcomes, there is no way to determine the effect of an intervention. Measurement is also the foundation on which the continuous quality improvement process is built. However, measurement of disease management systems is often complex, and flawed evaluation processes result in disputed outcomes. In this chapter, we will review how to plan the process of measuring outcomes of disease management interventions; from determining what outcomes to measure through identifying the appropriate measurement methodology. We will provide a general overview of methods and tools used to assess the value of disease and health management initiatives. This chapter should help you to

- Understand the importance of evaluating various interventions and their impact on optimizing care

- Understand the factors that determine health care value and quality and the methods used to measure them in practice

- Design and implement assessments of disease management initiatives within the health care setting

Why Measure Disease Management Interventions?

The soaring costs of health care have led to increased attention on measures to control expenditures and improve the quality of care in the United States (Toscani and Patterson, 1995; Relman, 1998). This new focus is not a sudden development but the result of an evolutionary process—our health care system moved through eras of expansion (the 1940s through the 1960s) and cost containment (the 1970s through the 1990s) before turning its emphasis to outcome assessment and accountability. All individuals involved with providing health care interventions must now be active participants in evaluating the value of their services to their consumers. Outcomes research has grown dramatically in recent years through the multidisciplinary efforts of epidemiologists, economists, statisticians, psychologists, sociologists, ethicists, and health service researchers and providers (Epstein and Sherwood, 1996). Drivers of this interest have been stimulated by years of growing health care costs, the emergence of the consumer as a key player in medical decisions, and the building of information systems to measure the cost and quality of services provided.

Disease management is a relatively new concept that has emerged as a result of the changing health care environment. Although many definitions exist, most would agree it involves a systematic process to identify, treat, and monitor populations of individuals with or at risk for disease with the continuous goal of optimizing care and cost (Todd, Eichert, and Toscani, 1985). Key elements at the core of disease management are the principles of outcomes research and health care value.

Health care value (HCV) has a variety of forms. Understanding the concept and its components is important in structuring and measuring the impact of interventions on our health care system. In the field of economics, value has historically been characterized as the ratio of utility to cost:

$$\text{Value} = \frac{\text{Utility}}{\text{Cost}}$$

In contrast, HCV has been defined as the ratio between out-come and cost, where the term *outcome* includes clinical benefit, satisfaction, and quality of life:

$$HCV = \frac{Outcome}{Cost}$$

or:

$$HCV = \frac{Clinical\ outcome + satisfaction + health\text{-}related\ quality\ of\ life}{Cost}$$

In the final HCV equation, satisfaction is defined as perceived satisfaction on the part of the health plan member, patient receiving care, payer, provider, or any combination of these. Health-related quality of life is the impact of overall health or disease on an individual's general well-being.

In reality, value can be very difficult to quantify because each component—clinical outcome, satisfaction, health-related quality of life, and costs—is defined based on differences in systems of measurement, availability of data collected, and perspective of the evaluator. Different units of measurement apply to each utility measured, making it very difficult to quantitatively compare the impact of different therapies or disease management interventions on health care value. Nonetheless, from a conceptual standpoint, value is an important qualitative determinant in health care decision making. Measuring and managing outcomes are central to this concept.

Through this discussion of health care value, we have been able to answer the critical question of why we should measure disease management interventions. The remainder of this chapter will focus on answering several other key questions, including:

- What should be measured?

- How should outcomes of the intervention be measured?

- When should the outcomes be measured?

What Should Be Measured?

Outcome measures take three forms: clinical, economic, and humanistic. Although all three types of outcomes ideally would be considered in any resource allocation or clinical decision making, this is not always possible or practical. Depending on the research perspective, outcomes of interest will vary.

Clinical outcomes are medical events such as rates of infections, myocardial infarctions, migraine attacks, or strokes. Intermediary end points can be used to describe and quantify the predictability of clinical outcomes (blood pressure measurements for stroke, cholesterol readings for heart disease, and CD_4 counts for infection rates in HIV patients). *Economic outcome measures* include the direct and indirect costs of delivering overall care and treating the disease (such as medications, office visits, hospitalizations, surgeries, and productivity loss). Examples of *humanistic outcomes* include health-related quality of life, functional status, patient preferences, and patient satisfaction. These measures are particularly important to plan members, patient caregivers, and employers.

Examples of the three distinct types of outcomes and some advantages and disadvantages of each are seen in Table 8.1.

In addition to evaluating these types of outcomes, health plans also measure structure and process variables of care. *Structure variables* are used to characterize the presence or absence of systems and facilities that are necessary for high-quality health care. *Process variables* reveal how health care delivery mechanisms affect patient outcomes (Holdford and Smith, 1997).

Examples of structure variables are the number of available providers and specialists, their location, and the tools used to monitor therapy. Process variables may include number of tests ordered, number of medications switched or changed, and the number of specialty referrals to other health professionals.

Disease management providers commonly make the decision to measure intermediate end points, sometimes referred to as *surrogate*

Table 8.1.   Advantages and Disadvantages of Specific Outcome Types.

Outcomes	Examples	Advantages	Disadvantages
Clinical	Death, stroke, heart attack, cure	Not intrusive, meaningful	Observation influenced by confounding factors; outcomes may be too long-term to measure
Economic	Hospitalizations, clinic visits, labs, work loss, ER visits, medications	Accounts for cost	Difficult to determine all relevant costs; debate surrounding methodology and cost identification
Humanistic	Quality of life, functional status	Patient centered	Patient burden confounders

Source: Adapted from Motheral, 1997.

end points, that do not adequately measure the true benefits of the program. It may be tempting to measure surrogate end points for a number of reasons, including when the desired outcome is not readily obtained with available data or when the outcome may not be observed for several years. Despite these obstacles, disease management providers should strive to avoid poorly represented surrogate end points because administrative or regulatory bodies may dismiss such outcomes as insufficient.

Examples of diseases that are often measured by evidence-based surrogate end points are seen in Table 8.2. In each of these cases, the surrogate outcome has been used as an indicator of the development or risk of the desired outcome.

How Should Outcomes Be Measured?

One of the most critical issues to consider before initiating a disease management program is the mechanism for measuring the effect of the intervention. In today's competitive managed care marketplace, allocating resources toward the measurement process may be extremely challenging. Although the initiative itself may reduce resource consumption, health care administrators may require that these reductions exceed the cost of program development, implementation, and monitoring.

Efficacy Versus Effectiveness

The difference between efficacy and effectiveness research is important in evaluating disease management interventions. Efficacy studies, for the most part, are conducted by specialized practitioners treating selected patients following a protocol in a controlled setting that is unlike clinical practice. Effectiveness studies, on the

Table 8.2. Desired Versus Surrogate Outcomes for Selected Diseases.

Disease	Desired Outcome	Corresponding Surrogate Outcome Measure
Coronary artery disease	Reduced incidence of myocardial infarction	Cholesterol or blood lipids
Hypertension	Reduced number of thromboembolic events	Blood pressure
Diabetes	Reduced long-term complications	HbA_{1c}
Asthma	Reduced number of symptoms or attacks	Increased inhaled steroid usage
		Decreased beta agonist usage
HIV/AIDS	Degree of advanced disease	CD_4 count

other hand, are relatively uncontrolled and take place in usual care settings (Epstein and Sherwood, 1996; Brooks and Lohr, 1985). Table 8.3 compares the characteristics of each type of study.

Most effectiveness studies are observational in that groups are not randomly selected for a particular therapy or observed for relevant outcomes over time. Selection bias, which occurs when patients are not randomly assigned to alternative treatments, is a problematic issue in this instance and adjustments for case mix and illness severity must be considered. As a result, a number of prospective effectiveness trials have risen in the past several years that include a pretrial hypothesis, protocol, informed consent, randomization, and timed data collection procedures. Unlike clinical trials, these studies enroll heterogeneous patient groups and are conducted in typical practice settings. Protocol, entry criteria, and

Table 8.3.   Effectiveness Studies Versus Efficacy Studies.

Criterion	Efficacy Studies	Effectiveness Studies
Study design	Randomized, blinded, controlled	Observational with or without blinding or controls
Patient population	Homogenous	Heterogeneous
Patient entry	Tightly controlled	Consecutive
Informed consent	Required	May or may not be necessary depending on nature of intervention and organization policies
Treatment	Comparison with placebo or other intervention	Comparison with usual care
Provider	Experienced investigator, academic medical center	Usual caregivers
Outcomes	Clinical end points	Patient outcomes
Generalizability	Limited	Broad

Source: Modified from Epstein and Sherwood, 1996.

other controls are kept to a minimum to mimic daily practice and outcome measures are carefully selected to answer key questions regarding treatment effects in these settings.

Although effectiveness studies are not controlled per se, it is important to include a comparison group that does not receive the intervention so that changes that occur due to the health care environment and natural changes do not confound results. This is one of the major criticisms of early disease management programs, which touted decreases in utilization resulting from an intervention in the absence of data describing utilization in patients who *did not* receive the intervention. Therefore, we recommend that each outcomes research initiative be carefully planned to ensure use of the most appropriate study method available for the given objectives and resources.

Study Design

Choosing a study design involves evaluating sources of available data and weighing the costs and consequences of each design. There are three general types of study designs that may be employed: retrospective, prospective, and models, as shown in Figure 8.1. As a rule, the studies are correlational; that is, they are centered on demonstrating a relationship between the intervention and observed outcome(s).

In a *retrospective study,* the evaluation is initiated after the outcomes have been observed. Therefore, data are exclusively historical in nature and could be subject to the influence of confounding factors. Retrospective studies include database analyses and chart reviews.

Prospective studies involve selecting one or more cohorts of patients and following them for the observed outcome(s) over time. The degree of randomization and control must be determined prior to initiating the study with the caveat that implementing these factors within the study may reduce researchers' ability to extrapolate results to a larger, more diverse population.

Figure 8.1.   Types of Outcome Studies.

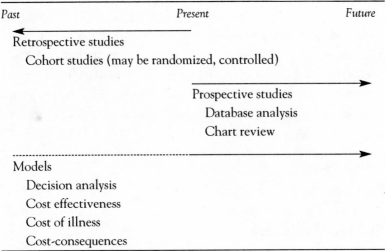

Outcomes research modeling is a useful approach when the primary study objective is to predict the future effect of an intervention on outcomes and ability to collect prospective data is limited. In this type of study, retrospective data such as results of database analyses and prior efficacy or effectiveness studies are used to model the potential effects of an intervention over time. Types of models include decision analyses ("decision trees"), cost effectiveness, cost-consequence, and cost of illness analyses. Although these designs are relatively inexpensive and quick to complete, the quality of input data must carefully be considered because it has a significant impact on study results.

Accounting for External Influences

One of the major criticisms of using select outcomes as indicators of the quality of care is that lack of study controls increases the likelihood that results are confounded by external influences. Before deciding how each outcome will be measured, potential influences must be considered. Is the outcome a factor of the intervention itself or of other variables (diet, lifestyle, or environment)? If possible, disease management providers should measure these factors in addition to the outcomes of interest. For example, a diabetes program including HbA_{1c} as an outcome to be measured should also include a survey of diet, self-care, and compliance before and after the initiative. In another example, an asthma program evaluation should include measurement of environmental changes. By recognizing and accounting for these influences, quality and credibility of program results are enhanced.

Data Sources

Claims data are a convenient and relatively inexpensive source of outcomes data. Managed care organizations maintain four primary types of internal databases:

- Medical claims data

- Pharmacy claims data

- Member eligibility data

- Provider data

Before initiating the baseline assessment, it is important to evaluate the contents of available internal databases. What data fields are included? Are the fields available for patients receiving care throughout the organization or just for certain divisions, for instance, outpatient, inpatient, radiology, blood bank, or specialty clinics?

Medical and pharmacy claims databases were originally designed as a means to bill for services rendered to patients. As such, they include demographic and utilization data but provide a limited depth of clinical data. Patient diagnoses, office visits, and prescription history are three clinical parameters that are typically included within these databases. Member eligibility databases contain coverage history as well as patient demographics. Provider databases may be of benefit for corresponding with specific physicians or practices, although content is limited to physician identifier codes, DEA license numbers, and personal information (addresses and phone numbers).

Many public data sources are also available through federal, state, and local agencies. The National Center for Health Statistics maintains many of the federal databases, and these may be accessed free of charge on the World Wide Web through FEDSTATS (www.fedstats.gov). A listing of some of the health-related databases is shown in Exhibit 8.1.

Exhibit 8.1.   Selected Federal Health Databases.

Centers for Disease Control and Prevention, National Center for Health Statistics (www.cdc.gov)
    National Vital Statistics System (NVSS)
    National Health Interview Survey (NHIS)
    National Health and Nutrition Examination Survey (NHANES)
    National Ambulatory Medical Care Survey (NAMCS)
    National Hospital Ambulatory Medical Care Survey (NHAMCS)
    National Nursing Home Survey (NNHS)
    National Immunization Survey (NIS)
    National Survey of Family Growth (NSFG)

Agency for Health Care Policy and Research (www.ahcpr.gov)
    HIV Cost and Services Utilization Study (HCSUS)
    Medical Expenditure Panel Survey (MEPS)
    Healthcare Cost and Utilization Project (HCUP)

Food and Drug Administration (www.fda.gov)
    MedWatch Database (national reporting system of adverse drug events)

Health Care Financing Administration (www.hcfa.gov)
    Medicare Provider Analysis and Review-MEDPAR (all inpatient
      visits for Medicare patients)
    National Claims History File (for Medicare, parts A and B)

Bureau of the Census (www.census.gov)
    National Census
    Economic Census

Source: FEDSTATS (2000).

Surveys

Although claims databases may be the most convenient and inexpensive source of outcome data, humanistic parameters must be measured through patient surveys (McGuire, 1996). In addition, patient surveys are useful for measuring clinical outcomes for certain diseases with intangible or subjective symptomatology, including depression and pain. Disease management providers must therefore understand potential patient and survey bias inherent in self-reported data obtained from questionnaires and would do well to use validated instruments.

Survey Types

The two primary types of surveys available to disease management providers are general and disease specific. General surveys assess the overall health status and well-being of the patient. Some commonly accepted tools include Medical Outcomes Study Short Forms 36 and 12 (SF-36 and SF-12), AAHP Satisfaction Battery, Sickness Impact Profile (SIP), and Activities of Daily Living (ADL) scale. These instruments would be useful in demonstrating the value of a dietary or fitness program but would fall short in measuring outcomes peculiar to specific conditions.

Disease-specific instruments are useful when specific data regarding a patient's illness are needed. A complete listing of such tools was compiled by Berzon, Simeon, Simpson, and Tilson (1993), although instruments continue to be developed through new research. Often, disease-specific tools are of more value to disease management providers because questions may directly assess the outcomes targeted by the disease management intervention. For example, the effects of a depression program could be measured by the Beck Depression Inventory or the Hamilton Depression Scale.

Survey Methodology

Before selecting an instrument to measure the intervention, the team should discuss the following factors:

1. Length of the questionnaire

2. Question format

3. Survey reliability and validity

4. Method of administration

The length of the questionnaire is a key consideration when choosing a measurement tool. Whether the respondent is a patient or clinician, time is of the essence, and limiting the time requirement will improve both the number and quality of the responses. Some of the key questions that must be addressed include:

- How much time will the respondent have to complete the assessment?

- If the survey is for the patient, will it be administered during an office visit or at home?

- Will the patient be mentally and physically able to complete the questionnaire?

- Does the language and educational reading level fit the population of interest?

- If the survey is clinician administered, will it be completed during an office visit or during other work time?

The format of survey questions is also a factor in survey response. Open-ended questions generally force the respondent to complete a thought or series of ideas. Although the responses obtained are likely to be thorough, it will probably be difficult to analyze them and draw conclusions about large sample populations. When possible, researchers should select tools with multiple-choice or rating-scale type questions or both. Multiple-choice, also known as multiple-guess, questions force the respondent to choose one of a series of potential responses. The respondent would have to decide which "bucket" his response best fits into and then select that choice.

In contrast, rating-scale questions force the respondent into weighting the degree of a certain outcome. In this way, rating-scale questions allow continuous variables to be assessed as categorical data. For example, pain may be thought of as ranging on a continuous spectrum from mild to severe, which may be assessed by a rating scale that ranges from 1 (mild pain) to 10 (severe pain). Most commonly used instruments include this format because categorical data enhance the ability to analyze the responses. In addition to this, these question types inherently lend themselves to improved accuracy of response.

The third consideration in selecting the instrument is its reliability and validity. The reliability of an instrument refers to the reproducibility of the response. Is the information the result of true signals or just background variability that occurs with that condition? If the variability between responses is much greater than the variability within responses from different patients, the instrument is said to be reliable. The measurement tool that is chosen should also have been validated in a study population comparable to that in the disease management evaluation. Validity indicates that the scale measures what it is supposed to measure (Holdford and Smith, 1997). *Content validity* refers to how completely the tool measures the outcomes it was intended to measure; *construct validity* indicates how well the survey measures predicted relationships between the outcome assessed and other variables.

The methods commonly used to administer surveys are mail, telephone, and live interview. Regardless of the mode selected, to obtain the optimal number and quality of response, respondents must understand how responding to the survey will benefit them. To accomplish this, the benefit of the information to respondents should be explained prior to administering the assessment.

From the perspective of a disease management provider, there are several considerations in selecting the appropriate patient survey administration method. These factors include expected response rates, potential for misunderstanding the questions, potential for missing items, cost, and turnover time. It is important to recognize that these factors are highly variable and depend on how the survey is designed and administered as well as the characteristics of the target audience.

The response rate will depend on the topic of the study, the interviewer and interviewing environment and media, and incentives offered. For example, a mail survey about asthma may have a greater response rate than one about sexually transmitted disease. Further, a mail survey about sexually transmitted disease may have a greater response rate than a telephone interview because of patient embarrassment. The general range of response rates has been reported to be 30 to 40 percent for mail surveys and 40 to 50 percent for telephone surveys; live interviews are likely to have a greater response rate than either of these options (Armstrong and Manuchehri, 1997). Further information regarding response rate can be found in the article by Hall (1995) in the Additional Resources section at the end of this chapter.

The potential for misunderstanding questions and missing items are two related factors, particularly in the case of mail surveys. If the questions are not constructed in a clear and concise manner, patients may not understand how to respond and therefore be reluctant to complete such items. In the case of telephone and on-site interviews, the interviewer's knowledge and technique will play a role in question understanding and, in turn, quality of response. For these reasons, it is always beneficial to conduct a pretest of survey materials and ensure that interviewers are similarly trained.

Cost and turnaround time are two other important considerations. Mail surveys are less expensive than telephone or on-site interviews, but they generally take longer to administer. These factors will need to be weighed in relation to the time and resources allocated to conducting the assessment.

Data Collection Systems

Managed care providers must consider the relative advantages and disadvantages of manual versus electronic data collection systems. The choice should depend on the breadth, depth, and scope of end points to be collected. For baseline assessments and pilot programs, manual systems are usually adequate because the amount of data is typically small. However, electronic data-capture systems may be required for large-scale assessments. These systems may be web based or incorporate interactive voice response technology. In some circumstances, the outcomes of interest can be measured exclusively via claims data, thereby avoiding the issue of choosing a system.

Regardless of the choice in system, it is important that the assessment tool be reviewed by several members of the disease management team before initiation of the pilot. Two of the questions that must be answered at this point are:

- Does the assessment measure the outcomes that the program was designed to improve?

- Will it be financially and mechanically feasible to collect the end points of interest using the chosen system?

If the data collection system meets these requirements, it should be pretested using mock data. For example, surveys can be administered to a few team members or patients, and claims data can be tested by requesting a preliminary report of patients with the diagnosis and parameters of interest.

When Should Outcomes Be Measured?

Determining when to measure the impact of the intervention seems simple relative to other considerations, but it can have a dramatic impact on the plausibility of results. Most often data collection time points are determined by the natural course of the disease itself. For example, measuring the impact of an influenza intervention may require identifying flu episodes during winter months and assessing the outcomes related to a five- to seven-day period associated with each. In contrast, a diabetes intervention may not necessitate measurement for six months to one year postimplementation because several months are required in order to observe measurable changes in long-term outcomes (such as HbA_{1c} levels and long-term complication rates).

Other factors that should be considered in deciding when to measure include the availability of human and nonhuman resources as well as organizational influences. Human resources include information technology personnel and biostatisticians. Nonhuman resources consist of hardware and software required to collect, extract, and analyze data. Organizational influences may also drive when measurement occurs, particularly when internal budgets dictate project timeliness or results are required for upcoming accreditation initiatives.

Case Study: Diabetes Disease Management Intervention

As a medical director of Healthy Care, a 200,000-member HMO with divisions in ten states, you have been offered a "new and innovative" diabetes program by an established disease management vendor. The program, called TotalControl, will cost $100,000 in start-up fees plus $400 for each Healthy Care patient with diabetes who is enrolled. The specific patient targets for the program are adults with either Type I or Type II diabetes. TotalControl includes the following:

- Provider education

    Continuing education program to educate Healthy Care's primary care physicians about the American Diabetes Association standards of care

    Laminated pocket cards that summarize these standards

- Patient education

    Brochures on diet, exercise, and self-monitoring

    On-line access to these educational materials

    Videotape on medication compliance

    Self-monitoring tools (glucometer, which electronically records blood glucose levels)

TotalControl is said to result in the following specific improvements in patient care and reduced utilization:

- Improved glycemic control through enhanced patient and provider compliance with guidelines

- Reduction in costs associated with the long-term complications (LTC) of diabetes, including nephropathy, neuropathy, and retinopathy

- Improved member satisfaction

- Improved provider satisfaction

Baseline Assessment

Before accepting TotalControl, you must determine whether or not the benefit of the program will exceed the cost to Healthy Care. An internal review of available demographic claims data using ICD-9 codes reveals that approximately 4,000 Healthy Care members are eligible for the program. To determine how many of these have Type I versus Type II diabetes, you assess ICD-9-CM data and confirm diagnoses with pharmacy utilization data.

In addition to the retrospective claims analysis, you conduct a prospective review of current practices. Through an informal telephone survey of primary care physicians (PCPs) at three Healthy Care group practices, you find

- No formal diabetes counseling or screening is taking place.

- No formal diabetes treatment guidelines are available to the practitioner.

- Physicians do not continually reinforce the importance of treatment and self-monitoring compliance.

- The average time spent per follow-up visit is approximately ten minutes.

Pilot

Based on the findings of the baseline assessment, it is decided to pilot TotalControl in three large PCP group practices. Three additional PCP group practices will participate as control sites, for comparison of intervention versus nonintervention patients. Providers are randomized to provide either the TotalControl intervention or usual care. The duration of the pilot is to be twelve months, with an interim assessment of 120 patients at six months. The outcomes measurement plan for the pilot is shown in Table 8.4. Results are shown in Table 8.5.

Intervention Quality Improvement

The postpilot assessment revealed that HbA_{1c} varied by demographic subpopulation. Based on these results, black females with Type I and Type II diabetes and white females with Type II were identified as subpopulations needing further improvement (see Table 8.6).

In response to this finding, Healthy Care added case management services to the TotalControl pilot. Specifically, the case managers were introduced to ensure patient compliance with diet, lifestyle, and medications for all patients with HbA_{1c} over 10.5 percent within target subpopulations. After enrollment in the pilot, participants received follow-up phone calls from their designated case manager every month for three months, then every other month thereafter.

Six months after implementation of the service, outcomes were reassessed. HbA_{1c} was shown to have been decreased to 7.7 percent; no change in the incidence of LTC was noted.

Table 8.4. Outcomes Measurement Plan for TotalControl Program.

Type	Outcome(s) of Interest	Data Used to Measure Outcome(s)	Data Source
Clinical	• Glycemic control	• HbA_{1c}	• Healthy Care's lab provider
	• Incidence of LTC • Process measures	• Tests ordered HbA_{1c}, foot exams, eye exams	• Healthy Care's claims data
Economic	• Hospitalizations • Outpatient visits • ER visits • Pharmacy utilization	• Reimbursement charges	• Healthy Care's claims data (medical and pharmacy)
Humanistic	• Member satisfaction • Provider satisfaction	• Satisfaction surveys	• Healthy Care's quality improvement department
	• Quality of life	• Survey (SF-12)	• Survey administered to diabetics by disease management team

Table 8.5.   Results of TotalControl Postpilot.

Type	Outcome	Indicator	Results
Clinical	Glycemic control	HbA_{1c}	9.5% (mean)
	Process measures	HbA_{1c} tests Number of foot and eye exams	Increase in HbA_{1c} measurements (10%) Increase in foot exams (5%) Increase in eye exams (5%)
Economic	Hospitalizations Outpatient visits ER visits Pharmacy utilization	Reimbursement	Outpatient visits increased by 20%
Humanistic	Member satisfaction	Satisfaction surveys	Slight increase in satisfaction
	Quality of life (QOL)	QOL survey	QOL remained about the same

Table 8.6.   Results After Implementing Case Management Component.

	HbA_{1c} (%) by Subpopulation			
	Type I		Type II	
	Female	Male	Female	Male
Black	9.8	8.5	9.8	8.0
White	9.2	8.0	10.0	8.4

Roll-Out

Based on the positive results of the pilot, it was decided to roll out the program for Healthy Care PCP group practices in five states. A reassessment was planned in six months, with subsequent roll-out to the remaining five states pending results from the first six months postimplementation.

Conclusion

In summary, measurement is a key aspect of any disease management system. It is required to demonstrate the value of the intervention to health care stakeholders, including payers, providers, and patients. Although stakeholders' definitions of value may differ based on their individual perspective, they are likely to consist of some balance of clinical, economic, and humanistic outcomes in relation to the cost of the intervention.

Measurement should be contemplated during the intervention development process. Researchers should establish outcome goals up front and consider how relevant parameters will be collected in order to demonstrate the intervention's value. Practical considerations include identifying an appropriate study design and instrument, determining data sources and data collection time points, and ensuring that resources needed to complete the measurement are available. These elements are required to successfully demonstrate the impact of the intervention and may serve to justify continued disease management efforts.

References

Armstrong, E. P., and Manuchehri, F. "Ambulatory Care Databases for Managed Care Organizations." *American Journal of Health System Pharmacy*, 1997, 54, 1973–1983.

Berzon, R. A., Simeon, G. P., Simpson, R. L., and Tilson, H. H. "Quality of Life Bibliography and Indexes." *Journal of Clinical Research and Drug Development*, 1993, 7, 203–242.

Brooks, R. H., and Lohr, K. N. "Efficacy, Effectiveness, Variations, and Quality: Boundary Crossing Research." *Medical Care*, 1985, 23, 710–722.

Epstein, R. S., and Sherwood, L. M. "From Outcomes Research to Disease Management: A Guide for the Perplexed." *Annals of Internal Medicine*, 1996, 124, 832–837.

FEDSTATS web site (www.fedstats.gov). 2000.

Holdford, D. A., and Smith, S. "Improving the Quality of Outcomes Research Involving Pharmaceutical Services." *American Journal of Health System Pharmacy*, 1997, 54, 1434–1442.

McGuire, G. "JCAHO Seeking to Play a Larger Role in MCO Accreditation." *Managed Care Outlook*, 1996, 9(5), 1–2.

Motheral, B. "Outcomes Management: The Why, What, and How of Data Collection." *Journal of Managed Care Pharmacy*, 1997, 3(3), 345–351.

Relman, A. S. "Assessment and Accountability—The Third Revolution in Medical Care." *New England Journal of Medicine*, 1998, 319, 1220–1222.

Todd, W. E., Eichert, J. H., and Toscani, M. R. "Disease Management—Building a Solid Foundation." *Disease Management and Health Outcomes*, 1985, 23, 710–722.

Toscani, M. R., and Patterson, R. B. "Evaluating and Creating Effective Patient Education Programs." *Drug Benefit Trends*, 1995, 7(9), 36–44.

Additional Resources

Bowling, A. *Measuring Health: A Review of Quality of Life Measurement Scales.* (2nd ed.) Bristol, Pa.: Open University Press, 1997, v–vii.

Eddy, D. *Assessing Health Practices and Designing Practice Policies: The Explicit Approach.* Philadelphia, Pa.: American College of Physicians, 1992.

Hall, M. F. "Patient Satisfaction or Acquiescence? Comparing Mail and Telephone Survey Results." *Journal of Health Care Marketing*, spring 1995.

McDowell, I., and Newell, C. *Measuring Health—A Guide to Rating Scales and Questionnaires.* New York: Oxford University Press, 1996.

National Committee for Quality Assurance. *Healthcare Quality Improvement Studies in Managed Care Settings.* Washington, D.C.: National Committee for Quality Assurance, 1994.

Spilker, B. *Quality of Life and Pharmacoeconomics in Clinical Trials.* (2nd ed.) Philadelphia: Lippincott-Raven Press, 1996.

. . . .

9

Selecting Variables and Constructs
to Measure

Joseph E. Biskupiak

The goal of this chapter is to review the major process and outcome constructs (measures) affected by health-related behavior management initiatives. The challenge in outcome measurement is to select those variables that are comprehensive, comparable, meaningful, and accurate in their representation of the effects of care (Kleinpell, 1997). First will be a review of outcome measurement in general and then a discussion of its application to health-related behavior management initiatives.

Outcome Measurement and Data Collection

In order to assess the quality of health care delivered to patients, it is imperative that the outcomes of care are measured. In our current competitive marketplace, these outcome measures are being used to compare all facets of health care. Outcomes are used to compare health plans, hospitals, individual providers, therapeutic interventions, and disease management programs.

For example, each year the Pennsylvania Health Care Cost Containment Council publishes the coronary-artery bypass graft surgery mortality rates for hospitals in the state (Anders, 1996). These mortality rates are prominently displayed by the media, and hospitals with high mortality rates engage in various forms of damage control. As this annual event clearly demonstrates, the measurement of outcomes of care is important and attracts much attention; however, there is considerable controversy over which specific outcomes should be measured and which methodology should be employed to measure them. The key issue that determines whether one chooses a specific process or outcome measure depends on the goals of the measurement process and the objectives of the intervention.

When engaging in outcome measurement, there are two types of data one can collect: process data and outcome data. Process data typically measure the rates of some aspect of health care utilization. Outcome data are representative of the clinical, humanistic (satisfaction and health-related quality of life), and economic results of therapeutic interventions (Schrogie, 1996).

Process Data

Process data measure the rates of preventive services and specific procedures. Process data are valuable because they are much easier to collect than outcome data. But process data have two major limitations in that they

- *Measure only the process of care*, which is related to the outcome of care in an indirect fashion

- *Are based on cross-sectional rather than longitudinal data* and provide no insight on what happens to a patient as a result of the treatment performed

For example, ABC Health Plan has a mammography screening rate (process data) of 85 percent for its eligible population, while the national average for health plans is 70 percent. This result could be interpreted as an example of ABC Health Plan's commitment to preventive care. Unfortunately, the reader has no idea about the breast cancer survival rate (outcome data) that results from ABC's diligent mammography screening program. When choosing a health plan, one would want to know not only the mammography screening rate but also the breast cancer survival rate of the health plan to make a truly informed choice.

Outcome Data

As previously mentioned, outcome data describe the clinical, humanistic, and economic results of therapeutic interventions. Outcomes are commonly grouped into three general categories:

- *System-centered clinical outcomes*, which reflect the clinical results and performance of therapeutic interventions, services, and products provided by health care providers

- *Patient-centered outcomes*, which describe the effect of a therapeutic product or service on how patients perceive their health status and satisfaction with care

- *Cost outcomes*, which include the use of resources associated with the administration of a product or service in a health care system (Schrogie, 1996)

An alternative view of outcomes considers the perspective of the entity interested in the outcomes. In this framework, outcomes are grouped by provider, patient, and payer (Kleinpell, 1997). There may also be occasions when it is appropriate to consider the perspective of the employer as distinct from the payer. Regardless of the framework one is most comfortable using, the goals of the measurement process need to be succinctly expressed such that the outcomes measured will allow one to assess the care delivered against those stated goals.

Exhibit 9.1 lists some commonly encountered outcome measures. Some of the measures may be considered as evidence of the quality and outcomes of clinical care (for example, rehospitalization rates). Other measures, typically those used to describe a drug's pharmacological effect, are surrogate end points and do not represent a long-term clinical outcome (such as blood pressure).

Exhibit 9.1.   Examples of Outcome Measures.

Nosocomial infection rates	Blood pressure
Adverse events due to drugs or devices	Social functioning
	Physical status
Postsurgical wound infection rates	Mental health status
Unanticipated returns to surgery	Worker productivity
Appropriateness of pain management therapies	Mobility and ambulation
Rehospitalization rates	Waiting time to obtain a physician appointment
Medication compliance	Length of stay
Hemoglobin A_{1C} levels	Cost of care
Cholesterol level	

Surrogate end points are important because they serve as an immediate indicator that allows one to assess whether change is occurring in a desired direction. Surrogates are useful measures when the desired outcome is not readily obtained with available data or when they may not be observed for several years (Weintraub, 1997).

For example, blood pressure is commonly measured as a surrogate end point in hypertension, in which the desired outcome one would like to be able to measure is the reduction in the number of thromboembolic events.

This very brief review of outcomes management in general leads us next to the application of outcome measurement in patient behavior change initiatives.

Outcome Measurement in Behavior Management Initiatives

As discussed in earlier chapters, the goal of health-related behavior management initiatives is to change and reinforce desired behavior and lifestyles that are expected to have a positive impact on chronic illnesses. Although our health care system has always focused on acute and episodic care, attention to chronic illness and its treatment has recently been recognized as an important component of our health care delivery system as we move into the new century (Strauss, 1987).

A study by Hoffman, Rice, and Sung (1996) determined the prevalence of chronic illness in the U.S. population and the total medical costs associated with treating patients with chronic conditions. It was determined that in 1987 there were ninety million Americans (37 percent of the total population) living with chronic conditions (total U.S. population 242.8 million). The authors estimate that, in 1995, there were almost 100 million Americans (38 percent of the total population, 263.2 million) living with chronic illness. In 1987, the costs of health services and supplies for non-institutionalized persons with chronic conditions totaled $272.2 billion, which accounts for 76 percent of the direct medical care costs (total $357.9 billion) in the United States in 1987 for noninstitutionalized persons. They also estimated 1990 health care costs for all persons with chronic conditions, which includes nursing home care costs, to be $425.2 billion, accounting for 64.5 percent of total 1990 health care costs ($659.5 billion).

Realization of the impact of chronic illness on our health care system has fueled the growth of a plethora of behavior management initiatives over the past several years. Health care organizations are faced with the daunting challenge of deciding which programs to offer to their covered population. Organizations need to be able to select those initiatives that have a positive impact on chronic illnesses.

In order to determine if these programs are successful, it will be necessary to evaluate them against their stated objectives. Evaluation presents several challenges for health care organizations and outcome researchers. It may be difficult to assess the impact of the initiative on patient health and functional status. This is particularly true when the short-term impact is being measured. In order to demonstrate differences, comparison with a control group is necessary (Christianson, Taylor, and Knutson, 1998). Rarely is there agreement on the appropriate control group and even if there is, such a group is unlikely to exist. Perhaps the biggest challenge, however, is that any evaluation process is going to be a costly endeavor. In spite of these challenges, it is important to recognize that providers, health care organizations, and purchasers will want to see that a credible assessment of an initiative's impact has been conducted. In addition, because behavior modification programs should be built on the foundation of continuous quality improvement, it will be necessary for the developers to maintain ongoing evaluation of the program's impact.

There are a variety of areas to consider when evaluating behavior change programs. Exhibit 9.2 lists many of the general areas that outcome measures should assess when evaluating programs.

Early evaluation efforts should focus on measures of patient satisfaction. It is unlikely that in the early phases of implementation there will be much data on process measures, health status, and clinical outcomes. Patient satisfaction is an outcome that can be influenced in the short term. It is also an outcome that health care organizations and providers need to consider in the short term, because without patient acceptance of the program, it is unlikely to succeed in the long term. As important in the early phases of implementation will be provider satisfaction. Both provider and patient satisfaction are likely to be correlated to the long-term acceptance and success of behavior initiatives (Christianson, Taylor, and Knutson, 1998).

Comparison (Control) Groups

As acceptance and utilization of a program increase, decision makers will want to know more about the program's impact on clinical and economic outcomes in addition to its impact on satisfaction. In order to assess the impact of the program, it will be necessary to compare its results to the results that would have been obtained in its absence. This will require an evaluation that includes a comparison (control) group that receives "usual care," that is, care in the absence of the program.

Exhibit 9.2.   Outcomes of Interest in Program Evaluation.
_____

Patient satisfaction
    Access to care
    Quality of care
    Functional status
    Physician interactions
    Ability to self-manage
    Patient education

Provider satisfaction
    Quality of care
    Ease of implementation and use of program
    Provider and patient education materials

Patient status
    Physical functioning
    Social functioning
    Psychological functioning
    Physiological parameters

Process measures
    Success of implementation efforts
    Participation rates in program for eligible patients and physicians

Economic measures
    Impact on direct medical costs
    Cost associated with program implementation and use
_____

Researchers and health care organizations have a couple of options for the construction of a control group. One option is to use the patients in the program as their own control group, comparing outcomes before inclusion in the program versus the outcomes achieved by participation in the program. There are two concerns with this approach. One issue is the appropriateness of comparing outcomes before and after the implementation of the program. As health care practice changes, is it realistic to say that care received prior to the program is the same as current practice received in the absence of the model? The other related issue deals with the length of time for the preimplementation evaluation period. Because most behavior change initiatives address chronic behavior, a long period is desirable to assess impact. A long preimplementation period, however, may not be advantageous for an organization eager to implement a new program. In order to leverage the early enthusiasm that the program has generated, it may be necessary to move forward quickly and enlist participants once the program is accepted. To avoid a long preimplementation data collection period, the program can be implemented immediately and a retrospective analysis of an administrative (claims) database conducted. The problem here is that only data captured in the database can be used for comparison purposes. Rarely does a database contain the measures necessary to fully evaluate a new program (Christianson, Taylor, and Knutson, 1998).

A second option is to create a control group of similar patients (a matched control group) that is receiving care at the same time as those that are participating in the program. Although this approach avoids the problems listed above, it presents a new set of problems. The challenge here is to identify a cohort of patients that have the same clinical characteristics as the treatment group and are receiving the same usual care minus the intervention program. If the health care organization has multiple providers caring for these patients, then randomization occurs at the provider level (that is, there are physicians participating in the program enrolling patients and their results are compared to physicians and their patients not participating in the program). The important question to consider is, are differences seen in the outcomes of the two patient groups attributable to the program or to differences in the care delivered by different providers? It may also be difficult for the health care organization to pilot the program with selected providers if all were involved in the adoption (buy-in) process. If the organization has invested considerable resources in convincing its providers of the value of the program, then the organization's ability to withhold its use by all may be limited. In order to avoid this political trap, the organization may be tempted to go outside its patient population to construct a control group. This is an unrealistic alternative because it will be very difficult to enlist patients and providers from outside the organization to obtain the necessary data (Christianson, Taylor, and Knutson, 1998).

Responsibility for Data Collection and Analysis

Once the organization has decided on the appropriate control group and measures to assess the program, it will be important to decide who will be responsible for data collection and analysis. The choices facing the organization are to conduct the work internally or to seek a credible external organization to conduct the analysis.

There are pros and cons associated with both internal and external review. The decision to seek external assistance may be driven by how the evaluation will be used or by whether or not the necessary expertise resides within the organization. If the need for program assessment is driven by internal needs regarding decisions to continue the program or modify the program (a continuous quality improvement activity), then internal review is appropriate, assuming the necessary expertise resides within the company. If the purpose of the program assessment is to satisfy the needs of those external to the organization (purchasers), a review conducted by an external organization may be deemed more credible than a self-evaluation. The concern of those health care organizations that enlist an external review is that they lose some control over the assessment. This can be mitigated to some degree by working with the external group during the assessment process (Christianson, Taylor, and Knutson, 1998).

For illustration purposes, let us now consider a hypothetical patient education program developed for asthmatics to improve their compliance with asthma medications. When constructing measures to assess the impact of a program, one needs to decide how to measure change and the relationship between the measure and the program's objectives. As stated earlier, change can be measured by either process or outcome measurements. This program's developers are trying to decide how they will demonstrate that the patient education intervention has resulted in an improvement in compliance with asthma medications. They have narrowed the list of possible measures to the following four:

1. *Asthma medication prescriptions.* Based on pharmacy data, it will be determined if asthmatics are obtaining their prescriptions in a timely fashion (a process measure).

2. *Asthma medication consumption.* Based on self-reported patient survey data or a patient diary, the frequency of medication usage will be determined (a process measure).

3. *Improvements in asthma symptoms.* Using either self-reported patient survey data or a patient diary, improvements in outcomes will be ascertained based on a reduction in the frequency of asthma symptoms (an outcome measure).

4. *Reductions in health care resource utilization.* Claims database analysis will be conducted to determine if there has been a reduction in resource utilization (an outcome measure).

In order to proceed, the developers need to consider the following two questions:

1. Does the assessment measure the outcomes that the program was designed to improve?

2. Will it be financially and logistically feasible to collect the end points of interest?

The patient education program was designed to improve compliance. Only the two process measures assess the intended objective of the education program. It is reasonable to assume that improved compliance with asthma medications will lead to improvements in the two outcome measures; however, the primary emphasis of the program was not reduction in asthma symptoms or resource utilization.

Evaluating the two process measures against the second question, the asthma medication prescriptions measure would appear to be the least costly and most feasible to collect. The pharmacy claims database could be used to determine refill rates for all patients in the education program. Actual medication usage derived from patient surveys has several problems. A survey instrument would be costly to develop and administer to patients, the dropout rate for responses to the survey will be high, and self-report data from patients can be unreliable. The developers should therefore consider the asthma medication prescriptions measure as their primary end point.

Self-Management Targets

The example above illustrates one of the tasks targeted by behavior change initiatives, namely, medication usage and compliance. There are several other process and outcome constructs that are affected by health-related behavior management initiatives. A review of patient education and self-care literature by Clark and others (1991) identified twelve self-management tasks that were routinely targeted across a variety of chronic diseases and conditions. The tasks identified are shown in Exhibit 9.3.

**Exhibit 9.3.   Self-Management Tasks Commonly Addressed in
Chronic Diseases and Conditions.**

1. Recognizing and responding to symptoms (including self-monitoring for symptoms and controlling triggers to symptoms)
2. Using medication
3. Managing acute exacerbations and emergencies
4. Maintaining good nutrition and an appropriate diet
5. Maintaining adequate exercise and physical activity
6. Quitting smoking
7. Using relaxation and stress-reducing techniques
8. Interacting appropriately with health care providers
9. Seeking information and using community resources
10. Adapting work and other role functions
11. Communicating with significant others
12. Managing the negative emotions and psychological responses to illness

Self-Management Measures

Lorig and others (1996) at the Stanford Patient Education Research Center developed a set of measures for use in chronic disease self-management programs that addresses the tasks listed in Exhibit 9.3 above. In addition to addressing self-management behavior and self-efficacy issues, it also has measures to address outcomes, particularly health status and health care utilization. These outcome measures, which are listed in Exhibit 9.4, are the result of the Chronic Disease Self-Management Program, a collaborative research study conducted by the Stanford University School of Medicine and the Kaiser Permanente Medical Care Program in northern California. A full description of each of the measures and references can be found in the book *Outcome Measures for Health Education and Other Health Care Interventions* (Lorig and others, 1996).

Putting Measurement Concepts into Practice

Up to this point, we have focused on the more theoretical aspects of measurement of health-related behavior management initiatives. Now let us turn our attention to some illustrative examples based on reports from the literature to see how researchers in the field have put into practice some of the concepts presented.

Obesity

Obesity is a potentially life-threatening disorder that is associated with an impaired quality of life and many comorbid conditions including diabetes, hypertension, congestive heart failure, coronary artery disease, and hyperlipidemia. Treatment recommendations for obese individuals typically include diet and exercise modifications to produce weight loss. These lifestyle changes frequently present a challenge for both the patient and provider. Health-related behavior management initiatives are frequently developed to address this challenge. It is important to recognize that obesity is a chronic disorder and, like other chronic disorders, interventions and outcome measurements need to focus on long-term, broad treatment outcomes. These broad treatment outcomes should include improved metabolic profiles, quality of life, psychological functioning, and physical fitness. This long-term focus presents a challenge to behavior change initiative development and outcome measurement.

A review by Foreyt and Poston (1998) examined the role of cognitive-behavior therapy (CBT) in obesity treatment. In obesity treatment, CBT consists of a methodology for modifying eating, exercise, and other behavior that are thought to contribute to obesity. The approaches to CBT in obesity include the use of self-monitoring and goal setting, stimulus control, and modification of eating style and habits—cognitive restructuring strategies that focus on challenging and modifying unrealistic or maladaptive thoughts, stress management, and social support.

Some of these approaches have implications for the types of outcomes that should be measured. For example, self-monitoring requires systematizing the observation and recording of behavior. Self-monitoring is important because research has shown that when individuals become more aware of their behavior and the factors that influence their behavior, treatment outcomes are improved. For obese individuals, self-monitoring may include the use of a diary to record eating and exercise activity as well as body measurements. Exhibit 9.5 lists some of the potential outcome measures recorded in the patient's diary.

The diary for obese individuals should also try to identify environmental cues that are associated with overeating and physical inactivity. Stimulus control attempts to modify these environmental cues and enable individuals to be successful at their weight loss activities. Almost all weight loss studies have recorded many of the outcomes mentioned above.

It is important to remember that there are also social and psychological components to obesity that CBT attempts to modify. In order for clinicians to engage obese patients in social restructuring, stress management, and social support programs, it will be important

Exhibit 9.4.   Chronic Disease Self-Management Program Measures.

Self-management behavior
    Stretching and strengthening exercise
    Aerobic exercise
    Cognitive symptom management
    Mental stress management and relaxation
    Use of community services for tangible help
    Use of community services for emotional support
    Use of community education and health support groups
    Use of organized exercise programs
    Communication with physician
    Advance directives
- Has living will and durable power of attorney
- Discussed with doctor
- Discussed with family

Self-efficacy
    To perform self-management behavior
- Exercise regularly
- Get information about disease
- Obtain help from community, family, and friends
- Communicate with physician

    To manage disease in general
    To achieve outcomes
- Do chores
- Attend social and recreational activities
- Manage symptoms
- Manage shortness of breath
- Control or manage depression

Outcomes
    Health status
    Disability
    Social or role activities limitations
    Pain and physical discomfort
    Energy or fatigue
    Shortness of breath

Exhibit 9.4.   *(continued)*

Psychological well-being or distress
Depressive symptoms
Health distress
Self-rated health
Health care utilization
- Visits to physicians
- Visits to mental health providers
- Visits to other providers
- Visits to emergency department
- Hospital stays
- Nights in hospital
- Outpatient surgeries

Source: Lorig and others, 1996.

Exhibit 9.5.   Patient Diary.

Eating diary	Exercise diary
Total caloric intake	Frequency
Calories from fat and fat grams	Duration
Food groups consumed	Intensity
Body measurements	
Weight	
Percentage of body fat	

for weight loss programs to also measure the psychosocial health status of obese patients. To date, very few weight loss programs have examined these outcomes. In order for behavior modification programs in weight loss to be successful, more attention will need to be given to this often overlooked component.

Although it is important to focus on the impact of behavior change initiatives on weight loss in obesity, weight loss should not be considered the only definition of treatment success. Improvements in other outcomes may also be regarded as indicators of a successful program. These outcomes include improvements in metabolic profiles (for example, lipids and glucose), exercise, self-esteem, quality of life, and functional status. Certainly weight loss is the ultimate goal of an obesity behavior change initiative. However, a program that results in a sedentary obese individual engaging in regular physical activity is beneficial. Exercise is associated with reductions in many comorbidities associated with obesity (Pate and others, 1995; Department of Health and Human Services, 1996). One study has demonstrated that regular exercise, even in obese men, significantly lowered age-adjusted risk of all-cause mortality compared with sedentary males (Barlow and others, 1995). This result indicates the importance of increasing physical activity levels and the benefits of exercise that can be achieved even if weight loss is not observed.

Hypertension

Hypertension is another area that is a frequent target of health-related behavior management initiatives. Hypertension is one of the most common forms of cardiovascular disease and it affects one in every four Americans (Intelihealth, 1998). The risk of having hypertension increases with age; 54 percent of people older than sixty have hypertension and 66 percent of people age 70 or older have high blood pressure. High blood pressure is a risk factor for many forms of heart disease. Clinical studies have demonstrated the interrelationship between hypertension and stroke, heart disease, congestive heart failure, and kidney failure. Stress management, weight loss, physical activity, healthy nutrition, medication compliance, and lower cholesterol levels all have beneficial effects on hypertension.

Health-related behavior management initiatives for hypertension have observed a variety of outcomes consistent with the healthy lifestyle factors mentioned above in addition to cholesterol and blood pressure levels. As seen in obesity, the primary indicators of success are the "numbers" (cholesterol and blood pressure levels); however, these are not the only indicators of a successful program.

A behavior change initiative that has a positive impact on any of the risk factors associated with hypertension (stress, weight, exercise, or diet) should be considered a successful program because these are also risk factors for other cardiovascular diseases. Cholesterol levels and blood pressure may require the use of medications in those individuals who experience improvement in other outcomes but not these important numbers as a result of a behavior change program.

Diabetes

Diabetes is a chronic, complex metabolic disease that results in the inability of the body to properly maintain and use carbohydrates, fats, and proteins. Most people with diabetes (95 percent of all cases) have a form known as noninsulin-dependent diabetes, or Type II diabetes, which occurs more often in people over the age of forty. A less common form of diabetes, known as insulin-dependent diabetes, or Type I diabetes, tends to occur in young adults and children. In these cases the body produces little or no insulin. People with Type I diabetes must receive daily insulin injections. For the patient living with either type of diabetes, close attention to diet and exercise is required. In addition, diabetes may reduce a patient's quality of life (QoL). The Diabetes Control and Complications Trial demonstrated that intensive therapy (tight glycemic control) provides the best protection from the long-term complications of diabetes (neuropathy, retinopathy, and nephropathy).

Health-related behavior management initiatives are frequently designed to target diabetic patients. Outcomes measured include diet and exercise (as described for obesity above) as well as blood glucose levels (HbA_{1c}). QoL is another outcome measure of importance in behavior change studies in diabetes. A recent article reported on the effects of a behavioral intervention (coping skills training) on glycemic control and QoL in adolescents on intensive therapy (Grey and others, 1998). The addition of this training to intensive therapy was found to have a positive impact on the adolescents' metabolic control and their QoL when compared to intensive therapy alone. Another behavioral intervention study with adolescent diabetics reported on the positive impact of the behavior intervention on treatment adherence (insulin usage and glucose testing), disease knowledge, and the ability to manage stress associated with social interactions (Mendez and Belendez, 1997). Improvements in disease knowledge (for any disease category) need to be interpreted with care. Many studies report improvements in patients' knowledge of their disease without demonstrating positive changes in behavior. The study by Mendez and Belendez reported improvements in disease knowledge that were concurrent with positive changes in behavior (that is, treatment adherence and stress management).

Behavior change initiatives that result in a better informed patient without concomitant positive changes in behavior are of little value. Although the study by Mendez and Belendez did not demonstrate improvements in glycemic control, it should still be considered a successful program due to its positive impact on treatment adherence, stress management, and disease knowledge.

Asthma

Asthma is a chronic inflammatory disease that causes the airways to narrow. Between twelve and fifteen million Americans have asthma, and it is the leading cause of chronic illness in children, affecting five million under the age of sixteen. Asthma severity levels vary from intermittent to mild, moderate, and severe persistent and the disease has a variable impact on QoL. Asthma severity can be modified but not cured by long-term anti-inflammatory medications (Cochrane, 1996).

Noncompliance with asthma medications is a common cause of treatment failure and may lead to unnecessary emergency care and hospitalization (Weinstein, 1995). Adherence to therapeutic regimens is difficult and is affected by a number of factors. Patterns of compliance are variable; some patients take less than the prescribed amount of drug all the time, and others take their prescribed medication at the right dosage and frequency for a period of time and then take a "drug holiday." Not one single factor accounts for the variations in compliance, but typically the frequency and ease of drug administration, adverse effects (whether real or perceived), and psychosocial issues can all affect compliance.

Interventions relying solely on patient education to improve asthma disease knowledge do result in increased disease knowledge but have a variable impact on asthma management behavior and asthma morbidity and mortality (Rubin, Bauman, and Lauby, 1989). Successful strategies to improve compliance (and ultimately reduce asthma morbidity and mortality) result in interventions using some combination of skills training, education, patient self-management practices, and behavior modification. Outcomes of interest in these interventions typically include some measure of asthma morbidity and mortality (that is, asthma symptom–free days, emergency room visits, nocturnal awakenings, asthma severity, asthma exacerbations, medication usage, and so on) as well as asthma disease knowledge, metered-dose inhaler technique, and self-management behavior (use of peak flow meters, medication compliance, avoidance of asthma triggers, and so on) (Wilson and others, 1993).

Conclusion

This chapter first presented the practical and theoretical considerations involved in assessing the outcomes of health-related behavior management initiatives. The chapter then presented some examples of work done in the field for chronic diseases and conditions that are predominant in our society, namely, obesity, hypertension, diabetes, and asthma. Health-related behavior management initiatives may result in improvements in the physiological parameters associated with these conditions or diseases (weight loss, lower blood pressure, lower HbA_{1c} levels, and lung function, respectively).

Improvements in physiological parameters should not, however, be the only measure of the success of behavior change interventions.

Interventions that result in regular physical activity, improved stress management, smoking cessation, improved diet, and increased functional status are just a few of many desirable outcomes that may result from these programs. Any and all of these outcomes associated with improvements in lifestyle should also be considered as indicators of a successful program.

References

Anders, G. "Who Ends Up Paying Cost of Cut-Rate Heart Care?" *Wall Street Journal*, Oct. 15, 1996.

Barlow, C. E., and others. "Physical Fitness, Mortality, and Obesity." *International Journal of Obesity and related metabolic disorders*, 1995, 19(suppl 4), S41–S44.

Christianson, J. B., Taylor, R. A., and Knutson, D. J. *Restructuring Chronic Illness Management: Best Practices and Innovations in Team-Based Treatment*. San Francisco: Jossey-Bass, 1998.

Clark, N. M., and others. "Self-Management of Chronic Disease by Older Adults." *Journal of Aging and Health*, 1991, 3, 3–27.

Cochrane, G. M. "Compliance and Outcomes in Patients with Asthma." *Drugs*, 1996, 52(suppl 6), 12–19.

Department of Health and Human Services. *Physical Activity and Health: A Report of the Surgeon General*. Atlanta: Department of Health and Human Services, Centers for Disease Control and Prevention, National Center for Chronic Disease Prevention and Health Promotion, 1996.

Foreyt, J. P., and Poston, W. S., II. "What Is the Role of Cognitive-Behavior Therapy in Patient Management?" *Obesity Research*, 1998, 6(suppl 1), 18S–22S.

Grey, M., and others. "Short-Term Effects of Coping Skills Training As Adjunct to Intensive Therapy in Adolescents." *Diabetes Care*, 1998, 21(6), 902–908.

Hoffman, C., Rice, D., and Sung, H. Y. "Persons with Chronic Conditions: Their Prevalence and Costs." *Journal of the American Medical Association*, 1996, 276, 1473–1479.

Intelihealth, "High Blood Pressure (Hypertension)." Web site (www.intelihealth.com). Nov. 1998.

Kleinpell, R. M. "Whose Outcomes: Patients, Providers, or Payers?" *Nursing Clinics of North America*, 1997, 32(3), 513–520.

Lorig, K., and others. *Outcome Measures for Health Education and Other Health Care Interventions*. Thousand Oaks, Calif.: Sage, 1996.

Mendez, F. J., and Belendez, M. "Effects of a Behavior Intervention on Treatment Adherence and Stress Management in Adolescents with IDDM." *Diabetes Care*, 1997, 20(9), 1370–1375.

Pate, R. R., and others. "Physical Activity and Public Health: A Recommendation from the Centers for Disease Control and Prevention and the American College of Sports Medicine." *JAMA: Journal of the American Medical Association*, 1995, 273, 402–407.

Rubin, D. H., Bauman, L. J., and Lauby, J. L. "The Relationship Between Knowledge and Reported Behavior in Childhood Asthma." *Journal of Developmental and Behavioral Pediatrics*, 1989, 10(6), 307–312.

Schrogie, J. J. "Outcomes Assessment." In D. B. Nash and N. Johnson (eds.), *The Role of Pharmacoeconomics in Outcomes Management*. Chicago: AHA Press, 1996.

Strauss, A. "Health Policy and Chronic Illness." *Society*, Nov./Dec. 1987, 25, 33–39.

Weinstein, A. G. "Clinical Management Strategies to Main Drug Compliance in Asthmatic Children." *Annals of Allergy, Asthma, & Immunology*, 1995, 74(4), 304–310.

Weintraub, M. "Measurement." *Pharmacy and Therapeutics*, Nov. 1997, 22(11), 536.

Wilson, S. R., and others. "A Controlled Trial of Two Forms of Self-Management Education for Adults with Asthma." *The American Journal of Medicine*, 1993, 94(6), 564–576.

Afterword

. . . .

The Beginning of a Revolution

Richard Patterson

W e live in interesting times. A number of factors are converging to bring health management practices and health behavior change to the forefront. Recently, one of the largest national managed health care organizations announced publicly that it will no longer be able to contain costs through administrative processes and that the primary means of containing escalating costs in the future will be through disease management. Simultaneously, the proliferation of health sites on the Internet (by some accounts numbering over 20,000) combined with the dramatic increase in direct-to-consumer advertising of pharmaceutical products have brought an unprecedented amount of health information to consumers.

These changes have created both opportunities and challenges. People with chronic illnesses, or simply interest in a health area, can access information geared to virtually any level of knowledge, understanding, or background. They can participate in communities of like-minded individuals and share experiences and ideas. They can use services that help them track and monitor important biometric measurements, like serum glucose for diabetics or peak expiratory flow for asthmatics. On the horizon is the ability to communicate more effectively and efficiently with care providers via the Internet, from asking questions and receiving reminders to scheduling appointments for follow-up care. The information available can be excellent in quality and comprehensiveness. It can also be valueless or misleading. Unfortunately the public at large is too often ill-equipped to know the difference.

Providers of health care services—physicians, hospital systems, and managed care plans—are wrestling with how best to approach this new world. Some physicians are frustrated and dismayed by the need to spend valuable time dispelling misinformation patients obtain from the Internet or acceding to demands from patients for medications seen in television or magazine advertising. Physician adoption of the Internet has been slow, particularly for use in communicating with and educating patients. In an August 1999 survey of physician's Internet use conducted by the American Medical Association, 37 percent of physicians report using the Internet. However, only 28 percent of that group (or 10 percent of all physicians) report using the Internet for patient information and 7 percent of the group (or less than 3 percent of physicians) report using the Internet to communicate test results to patients. Interestingly, 27 percent of physicians using the Internet report putting up personal or practice sites for use by their patients or for marketing purposes (Liebman, 2000). Most health plans are investing in the Internet, with services ranging from provider and claims databases to on-line health encyclopedias, health risk appraisals, and lifestyle change information. We are looking toward the day when advanced telemedicine services can be provided cost effectively over the Internet—technologically facilitated virtual house calls.

These are the beginnings of a revolution in health care. The day may be close upon us when physicians, patients, and Internet-based services combine to achieve better communication. Patients will be empowered and motivated, have better access to health care services, and develop the skills and understanding needed for integrating treatment of illnesses and risk-reducing lifestyle changes to achieve a fuller, more rewarding life.

Reference

Liebman, M. "Physicians Weave a Pattern of Web Use." *Medical Marketing and Media*, Jan. 2000.

Index

. . . .

Printed in the United States
48578LVS00002B/34

SOCIAL SCIENCE LIBRARY

Manor Road Building

WITHDRAWN

Manor Road
Oxford OX1 3UQ

Tel: (2)71093 (enquiries and renewals)
http://www.ssl.ox.ac.uk

This is a NORMAL LOAN item.

We will email you a reminder before this item is due.

Please see http://www.ssl.ox.ac.uk/lending.html
for details on:

- loan policies; these are also displayed on the notice boards and in our library guide.

- how to check when your books are due back.

- how to renew your books, including information on the maximum number of renewals. Items may be renewed if not reserved by another reader. Items must be renewed before the library closes on the due date.

- level of fines; fines are charged on overdue books.

Please note that this item may be recalled during Term.

WITHDRAWN